Health for All Policies

Factors outside of healthcare services determine our health and this involves many different sectors. *Health for All Policies* changes the argument about inter-sectoral action, from one focusing on health and the health sector to one based on co-benefits – a 'Health for All Policies' approach. It uses the Sustainable Development Goals as the framework for identifying goals across sectors and summarizes evidence along two causal axes. One is the impact of improved health status on other SDGs, e.g. better educational and employment results. The other is the impact of health systems and policies on other sectors. The 'Health for All Policies' approach advocated in this book is thus a call to improve health to achieve goals beyond health and for the health sector itself to do better in understanding and directing its impact on the world beyond the healthcare it provides. This title is also available as Open Access on Cambridge Core.

Scott L. Greer is a political scientist and specialist in the comparative politics of health, with special interests in federalism, the European Union, health governance and social policy. His recent books include *Everything you always wanted to know about European Union health policy but were afraid to ask* (third edition, 2022); *Ageing and Health: The Politics of Better Policies* (2021); and *Coronavirus Politics: The Comparative Politics and Policy of COVID-19* (2021).

Michelle Falkenbach is a technical officer at the European Observatory on Health Systems and Policies main office in Brussels and Adjunct Clinical Assistant Professor in the department of Health Management and Policies at the University of Michigan. Her main area of research is on the health and care workforce, focusing primarily on ways to increase retention and recruitment efforts for this sector. Prior to joining the Observatory, Dr. Falkenbach was a post-doctoral research at Cornell University focusing on the impact of populist radical right parties on health and health systems.

Josep Figueras is the Director and cofounder of the European Observatory on Health Systems and Policies. In addition to WHO, he has served major multi-lateral agencies such as the European Commission or the World Bank and has worked as policy advisor in more than forty countries. He was Co-chair of the Scientific Advisory Board of the Monti Commission, and member of several governing, advisory and editorial boards including the governance board of the European Health Forum Gastein.

Matthias Wismar is Programme Manager at the Observatory based in Brussels. His work focuses on health policy, politics and governance, the health workforce, European integration and intersectoral action and the Sustainable Development Goals. He is developing studies, policy briefs, rapid responses and face-to-face dissemination and knowledge brokering formats.

European Observatory on Health Systems and Policies

The volumes in this series focus on topical issues around the transformation of health systems in Europe, a process being driven by a changing environment, increasing pressures and evolving needs.

Drawing on available evidence, existing experience and conceptual thinking, these studies aim to provide both practical and policy-relevant information and lessons on how to implement change to make health systems more equitable, effective and efficient. They are designed to promote and support evidence-informed policy-making in the health sector and will be a valuable resource for all those involved in developing, assessing or analyzing health systems and policies.

In addition to policy-makers, stakeholders and researchers in the field of health policy, key audiences outside the health sector will also find this series invaluable for understanding the complex choices and challenges that health systems face today.

List of Titles

Challenges to Tackling Antimicrobial Resistance: Economic and Policy Responses
Edited by Michael Anderson, Michele Cecchini, Elias Mossialos

Achieving Person-Centred Health Systems: Evidence, Strategies and Challenges
Edited by Ellen Nolte, Sherry Merkur, Anders Anell

The Changing Role of the Hospital in European Health Systems
Edited by Martin McKee, Sherry Merkur, Nigel Edwards, Ellen Nolte

Private Health Insurance: History, Politics and Performance
Edited by Sarah Thomson, Anna Sagan, Elias Mossialos

Ageing and Health: The Politics of Better Policies
Scott L. Greer, Julia Lynch, Aaron Reeves, Michelle Falkenbach, Jane Gingrich, Jonathan Cylus, Clare Bambra

Skill-mix Innovation, Effectiveness and Implementation
Edited by Claudia B. Maier, Marieke Kroezen, Reinhard Busse

Series Editors

Health *for* All Policies

The Co-Benefits of Intersectoral Action

Edited by

SCOTT L. GREER
University of Michigan

MICHELLE FALKENBACH
European Observatory on Health Systems and Policies

JOSEP FIGUERAS
European Observatory on Health Systems and Policies

MATTHIAS WISMAR
European Observatory on Health Systems and Policies

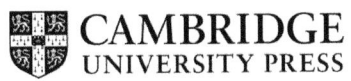

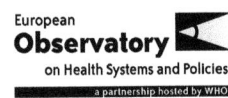

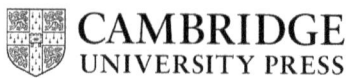

Shaftesbury Road, Cambridge CB2 8EA, United Kingdom

One Liberty Plaza, 20th Floor, New York, NY 10006, USA

477 Williamstown Road, Port Melbourne, VIC 3207, Australia

314–321, 3rd Floor, Plot 3, Splendor Forum, Jasola District Centre, New Delhi – 110025, India

103 Penang Road, #05–06/07, Visioncrest Commercial, Singapore 238467

Cambridge University Press is part of Cambridge University Press & Assessment, a department of the University of Cambridge.

We share the University's mission to contribute to society through the pursuit of education, learning and research at the highest international levels of excellence.

www.cambridge.org
Information on this title: www.cambridge.org/9781009467735

DOI: 10.1017/9781009467766

First published 2024

A catalogue record for this publication is available from the British Library

A Cataloging-in-Publication data record for this book is available from the Library of Congress.

ISBN 978-1-009-46773-5 Paperback

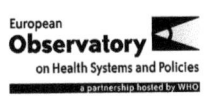

European Observatory
on Health Systems
and Policies

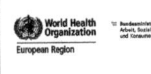 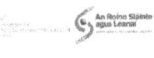

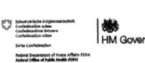   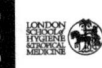

The European Observatory on Health Systems and Policies supports and promotes evidence-based health policy-making through comprehensive and rigorous analysis of health systems in Europe. It brings together a wide range of policy-makers, academics and practitioners to analyse trends in health reform, drawing on experience from across Europe to illuminate policy issues.

The European Observatory on Health Systems and Policies is a partnership hosted by the World Health Organization Regional Office for Europe, which includes the Governments of Austria, Belgium, Finland, Ireland, Kingdom of the Netherlands Norway, Slovenia, Spain, Sweden, Switzerland, the United Kingdom, and the Veneto Region of Italy (with Agenas); the European Commission; UNCAM (French National Union of Health Insurance Funds); the Health Foundation; the London School of Economics and Political Science; and the London School of Hygiene & Tropical Medicine. The Observatory has a secretariat in Brussels and it has hubs in London (at LSE and LSHTM) and at the Berlin University of Technology.

Contents

Figures

Tables

Boxes

Acknowledgements

In addition to the authors, who have engaged in developing the project and its central ideas, the editors would like to thank Martin McKee, Sebastián Peña, Peter C. Smith and Marc Suhrcke for their engagement and thoughts. We would also like to thank audiences at the European Health Management Association, European Public Health Association and Health Systems Global meetings for their helpful comments.

Contributors

Helena de Moraes Achcar has a PhD in International Relations from the London School of Economics. Her thesis focused on South-South cooperation between Brazil and Mozambique, where she did fieldwork to investigate the establishment of the first national pharmaceutical factory in sub-Saharan Africa, and an agricultural project called ProSavana. Her current research is about civil society's demand and mobilization (and demobilization) for universal access to treatment in Brazil. Her interests include public health, discourse analysis and South-South cooperation.

Jon Cylus is the head of the European Observatory on Health Systems and Policies' London Hubs based at both the London School of Economics and the London School of Hygiene and Tropical Medicine as well as a Senior Health Economist in the WHO Barcelona Office for Health Systems Financing and a Visiting Professor at the Barcelona Institute for Global Health (ISGlobal). His main research is on health systems, focusing primarily on health financing policy, health economics and health system performance. He has worked on these topics in a wide range of countries as well as with international organizations including the European Commission and OECD. Prior to joining the Observatory, Jon was an economist at the Centers for Medicare and Medicaid Services (CMS) in the United States where he worked on health care expenditure projections, hospital productivity, and health care expenditure estimates by age and gender.

Billy Dering is a Research Fellow at the Center on Health Insurance Reforms at Georgetown University. He has worked on projects with the European Observatory on Health Systems and Policies related to health financing. Billy previously worked in the U.S. Senate on health policy topics and on the health financing team at Epic Systems. He earned an MPH from the University of Michigan in the Department of Health Management and Policy, and a BA with distinction in Public

Policy from the University of Michigan. Billy previously worked in the U.S. Senate on health policy topics and on the health financing team at Epic Systems. He holds a BA with distinction in Public Policy from the University of Michigan, where he was awarded the Stamps Scholarship.

Michelle Falkenbach (PhD, University of Michigan) is a technical officer at the European Observatory on Health Systems and Policies main office in Brussels and a research associate in the department of Health Management and Policy at the University of Michigan. Her main area of research is on the health and care workforce, focusing primarily on ways to increase retention and recruitment efforts for this sector. Prior to joining the Observatory, Dr. Falkenbach was a post-doctoral research at Cornell University focusing on the impact of populist radical right parties on health and health systems.

Elize Massard da Fonseca is Associate Professor of Public Administration at the Getulio Vargas Foundation (Brazil), with years of experience researching pharmaceutical regulation in Latin America, health industry policy, and the politics of infectious diseases. Her publications have appeared in top journals such as the New England Journal of Medicine, Social Science and Medicine, and Research Policy; some were featured as the most downloaded (The political economy of Covid-19 vaccine regulation), most cited (The comparative politics of COVID-19), and with a higher score of attention (Coronavirus Politics). Her research, funded by FAPESP (#2021/06202–0), has proposed actions to improve access to pharmaceuticals in developing economies.

Scott L. Greer is a political scientist and specialist in the comparative politics of health, with special interests in federalism, the European Union, health governance and social policy. His recent books include *Putting Federalism in its Place: The Territorial Politics of Social Policy Revisited* (2023); *Everything you always wanted to know about European Union health policy but were afraid to ask* (third edition, 2022); *Ageing and Health: The Politics of Better Policies* (2021); *Coronavirus Politics: The Comparative Politics and Policy of COVID-19* (2021); and *The European Union after Brexit* (2021).

Iris Holmes, Cornell Institute of Host-Microbe Interactions and Disease

Holly Jarman is Associate Professor of Health Management and Policy and Global Public Health within the University of Michigan School of Public Health. As a political scientist, she compares health policies across countries and studies the impact of economic policies on health at the global level. She is the author of over 30 peer reviewed articles and several books on the governance of trade, tobacco products, pharmaceuticals, medical devices, and pandemic response. She also serves as Senior Social Scientist for the US Army Corps of Engineers, advising the US Federal government on comparative policy analysis and global pandemic response.

Ogujiuba Kanayo is currently an Associate Professor at the School of Development Studies at the University of Mpumalanga (UMP), South Africa. In the last three decades, Prof. Ogujiuba has played a significant role in cross-institutional collaboration and research, initiating activities furthering research development, and innovation activities. Before joining UMP, he was at the University of the Western Cape (UWC), South Africa between 2016 and 2019. Furthermore, Prof. Ogujiuba's understands indicators and information necessary to determine trends in counterfactual analysis and development policy. Additionally, Ogujiuba K. has built up solid relationships for academic collaboration between universities across the globe and supervises postgraduate students. He has published more than hundred (100) articles in peer-reviewed journals/conference proceedings/Technical Reports, in addition to more than fifteen (15) book chapters. He has been a policy advisor and team leader for several international agencies and a member of management committees throughout his career.

Jamison Koeman is the Program Manager of Housing Solutions for Health Equity at the University of Michigan and Public Health IDEAS for Creating Healthy and Equitable Cities at the University of Michigan School of Public Health. He is an expert on the intersection between housing and health and has published about health system investment in housing services. He has experience in eviction and foreclosure prevention work in Detroit and health policy work at the United States Government Accountability Office (GAO). Jamison received his MPH in Health Management and Policy from the University of Michigan School of Public Health.

Ellen Kuhlmann, PhD sociology, MPH, specialised nurse, is currently an interim Professor of Health and Health Systems care at the University of Siegen, Germany, and leading a project on migrant healthcare workers at Hannover Medical School as part of the German Global Health Research Alliance (GLOHRA) programme. Ellen is President of the European Public Health Association section 'Health Workforce Research' (EUPHA-HWR). She is researching health systems, policy and governance comparatively with a focus on the healthcare workforce, gender and intersectional inequalities, and COVID-19 policy.

Gabriela Lotta is a Professor of Public Administration at Fundação Getulio Vargas (FGV). She was a visiting professor at Oxford in 2021. She coordinates the Bureaucracy Studies Center (NEB). She is a professor at the National School of Public Administration, ENAP, a researcher at the Center for Metropolitan Studies (CEM), and in Brazil.Lab from Princeton University. Lotta received her B.Sc. in public administration and Ph.D. in Political Science at the University of São Paulo. In 2021 she was nominated among the most influential academics in the area of government.

Roshanak Mehdipanah is Associate Professor of Health Behavior and Health Education in the School of Public Health at the University of Michigan. Dr. Mehdipanah is Director of the Housing Solutions for Health Equity initiative and co-leads the Public Health IDEAS: Creating Healthy and Equitable Cities. She completed her PhD at the University of Pompeu Fabra, Spain. Her research is supported by grants from the National Institutes of Health, the Centers for Disease Control and Prevention and the World Health Organization, and focuses on the impact of urban policies, particularly related to the built environment, on health and health inequities of residents.

Marie Chantel Montás, Harvard University

Olaide O. Ojoniyi holds a doctoral degree in Population Studies. She is an Individual Consultant who recently completed a Census Thematic Analysis Report on Gender with the Pacific office of UNFPA. Her main research focus is on Adolescent girls and young women's sexual and reproductive health; Child and Maternal Health; Fertility and Equality. Over the years she has used quantitative methods to study these issues. She is currently exploring the computational method to study social and health issues. She won the 2016 Postgraduate merit award at the University of the Witwatersrand Johannesburg. She is a student member of the International Union for the Scientific Study of Population.

Janamarie Perroud, University of Michigan

Olivia Rockwell is a Global Health and Management graduate student at the University of Michigan's School of Public Health. She is a National Science Foundation Researcher and a Health Management and Policy Governance Lab Fellow. Previously, she was a Visiting Researcher for the European Observatory on Health Systems and Policies. She has been featured in an article in the BMJ and the recent European Observatory publication Health for All Policies.

Luigi Siciliani, Department of Economics and Related Studies at the University of York

Kristine Sørensen, Global Health Literacy Academy

Praneetha Vissapragada, University of Michigan

Gemma A. Williams is a Research Fellow at the European Observatory on Health Systems and Policies, and a PhD researcher in the Department of Social Policy, London School of Economics and Political Science. She conducts comparative health systems research, focusing primarily on the health and care workforce, health financing policy, health inequalities, healthy ageing, and digital health. Her work on these topics has been published in numerous peer reviewed articles, book chapters and policy reports. Gemma is co-editor of Eurohealth, the Observatory's quarterly journal. Gemma previously worked as a Research Officer at LSE Health and as an ODI Fellow Health Economist in the Rwandan Ministry of Health.

Charley E. Willison (PhD, University of Michigan) is an assistant professor of public health at Cornell University. She is a political scientist studying the relationships between local politics, intergovernmental relations, and public health political decision-making. Dr. Willison's 2021 book, Ungoverned and Out of Sight: Public Health and the Political Crisis of Homelessness in the United States (Oxford University Press) examines why municipalities may use evidence-based approaches to address chronic homelessness or not. Her book won the 2022 Dennis Judd Best Book Award, which recognizes the best book on urban politics (domestic or international) published in the previous year.

Abbreviations

ARV	Anti-retroviral
CBA	Cost-Benefit Analysis
CCMDD	Centralized Chronic Medicine Dispensing And Distribution
CHC	Continuing health care
CHD	Coronary heart disease
DCSTs	District Clinical Specialist Teams
DNDi	Drugs for Neglected Diseases initiative
ESIF	European and Structural Investment Funds
GAVI	Vaccine Alliance
GDP	Gross Domestic Product
GP	General Practitioner
GSPA-PHI	Global Strategy and Plan of Action on Public Health, Innovation and Intellectual Property
H4AP	Health for All Policies
HCW	Health and Care Worker
HCWF	Health and Care Workforce
HiAP	Health in All Policies
HPRS	Health Patient Registration System
HPV	Human Papillomavirus
ICRM	Ideal Clinic Realization and Maintenance Model
IPCC	Intergovernmental Panel on Climate Change

ISHP	Integrated School Health Programme
JOGG	*Jongeren op Gezond Gewicht* (Youth at a Healthy Weight)
LMIC	Low- and middle-income countries
MDG	Millenmium Development Goals
NDP	National Development Plan
NHI	National Health Insurance
ORAMMA	Operational Refugee and Migrant Maternal Approach
PDP	Productive Development Partenership
PHC	Primary Health Care
QALY	Quality-adjusted life years
R&D	Research and development
SAGMA	Southern African Generic Medicines Association
SDGs	Sustainable Development Goals
SMM	*Sociedade Moçambicana de Medicamentos* (Mozambican Pharmaceutical Ltd)
SSC	South–South cooperation
SVS	Stock visibility system
UHI	Urban Heat Island
UNCTAD	United Nations Conference on Trade and Development
WBPHCOT	Ward-based Primary Health Care Outreach Teams
WISN	Workload Indicator for Staffing Needs
WLPF	World Local Production Forum

1 From Health in All Policies to Health for All Policies: the logic of co-benefits

SCOTT L. GREER, MICHELLE FALKENBACH,
PRANEETHA VISSAPRAGADA, MATTHIAS
WISMAR

1.1 Introduction: beyond Health in All Policies

Everything affects health, but not everybody thinks health is their business. Health status and outcomes, it is known, are shaped by social, economic and political determinants as diverse as cigarettes, sewers and adult education. That argument has never been guaranteed to persuade interests and people who regard health as somebody else's problem. Sceptics might think that ill health is an individual failing, or something to be solved by hospitals and technology; or inevitable; or simply not a priority relative to some other goal such as fiscal rigour or How do we make the case for health?

Traditionally, health policy "advocates" have framed intersectoral collaboration as "Health in All Policies", though the impulse to work through other sectors to improve health far antedates the HiAP campaigns of the twenty-first century. HiAP arguments drew upon this widespread recognition that factors outside of health care services determine our health and that this involves many sectors (Ståhl et al., 2006). This understanding draws on arguments dating back to at least the Alma Ata Declaration (Chorev, 2012; Fukuda-Parr, 2018; Lawn et al., 2008; Weber, 2020) and many other documents, including the 2018 Tallinn Declaration (Cylus, Permanand & Smith, 2018). The COVID-19 pandemic and countries' responses to it has made the potential scope of a HiAP approach – of sorts – abundantly clear. During the pandemic, countries have implemented measures to prevent disease transmissions, adjust health systems, control borders and mobility, redirect the economy, and secure civil protection. In order to achieve this, many heads of government and their ministers of health worked closely with all other ministries (education, internal and foreign affairs, transport), departments (agriculture, research and state aid), and sectors (social affairs and transport) (Greer et al., 2022a; Sagan et al., 2021). We have also seen tremendous pressure to "return to normal", regardless of whether the epidemiological situation warrants it; the multiplicity of interests and goals in a modern society means that an all-out mobilization for any particular goal is politically unsustainable over time.

The volume of publications and policy attention dedicated to HiAP in global health debates is impressive. WHO's Helsinki Statement on Health in All Policies described HiAP as "an approach to public policies across sectors that systematically takes into account the health implications of decisions, seeks synergies, and avoids harmful health impacts in order to improve population health and health equity" (WHO, 2014). HiAP was the most important international movement to achieve health goals through intersectoral action. Health in All Policies is a "horizontal, complementary policy-related strategy contributing to improved population health. The core of HiAP is to examine determinants of health that can be altered to improve health but are mainly controlled by the policies of sectors other than health." (Ståhl et al., 2006; Box 1.1). HiAP entailed intersectoral governance or multi-sectoral governance, "coordinated action that explicitly aims to improve people's health or influence determinants of health. Intersectoral action for health is seen as central to the achievement of greater equity in health, especially where progress depends upon decisions and actions in other sectors." (Ståhl et al., 2006; Box 1.1).

Box 1.1 Definitions

Determinants of health refers to factors found to have the most significant influence – for better or worse – on health. Determinants of health include the social and economic environment and the physical environment, as well as the individual's particular characteristics and behaviours. Social and economic conditions – such as poverty, social exclusion, unemployment and poor housing – are strongly correlated with health status. They contribute to inequalities in health, explaining why people living in poverty die sooner and become sick more often than those living in more privileged conditions.

Social determinants of health can be understood as the social conditions in which people live and work. These determinants point to specific features of the social context that affect health and to the pathways by which social conditions translate into health impacts.

Health is, according to the official WHO definition, a state of complete physical, mental and social wellbeing and not merely the absence of

Box 1.1 (cont.)

disease or infirmity. Within the context of health promotion, health is seen as a resource for everyday life, not the object of living; it is a positive concept emphasizing social and personal resources as well as physical capacities.

Health promotion is the process of enabling individuals and communities to increase control over the determinants of health and therefore improve their health. It represents a strategy within the health and social fields which can be seen on the one hand as a political strategy and on the other hand as an enabling approach to health directed at lifestyles.

Health sector includes government ministries and departments, social security and health insurance schemes, voluntary organizations and private individuals, and groups providing health services.

Health in All Policies is a horizontal, complementary policy-related strategy contributing to improved population health. The core of HiAP is to examine determinants of health that can be altered to improve health but are mainly controlled by the policies of sectors other than health.

Intersectoral action for health could be defined as a coordinated action that explicitly aims to improve people's health or influence determinants of health. Intersectoral action for health is seen as central to the achievement of greater equity in health, especially where progress depends upon decisions and actions in other sectors. The term "intersectoral" was originally used to refer to the collaboration of the various public sectors, but more recently it has been used to refer to collaboration between the public and private sectors. The term **"multisectoral action"** has been used to refer to health action carried out simultaneously by a number of sectors within and outside the health system, but according to the WHO Glossary of Terms, it can be used as a synonym for intersectoral action.

Healthy public policy is, according to the Adelaide recommendations, "characterized by an explicit concern for health and equity in all areas of policy, and by an accountability for health impact. The main aim for healthy public policy is to create a supportive environment to enable people to lead healthy lives. Such a policy makes health choices possible and easier for citizens. It makes social and physical environment enhancing."

Public policy is policy at any level of government and may be set by heads of government, legislatures and regulatory agencies. Supranational institutions' policies may overrule government policies.

Source: Ståhl et al., 2006

Note how these definitions focus on what can be achieved for health by activities in other sectors. HiAP is an analytical tool and frame as a means to an end, which is healthy public policies (Kickbusch, 2010). The Adelaide Declaration called for "healthy public policy" that is "characterized by an explicit concern for health and equity in all policy areas, and by an accountability for health impact. The main aim for healthy public policy is to create a supportive environment to enable people to lead healthy lives. Such a policy makes health choices possible and easier for citizens. It makes social and physical environment enhancing." (Box 1.1).

The limitation of Health in All Policies thinking, as with many of the older social medicine and social determinants of health campaigns, is that it frames the issue in unidirectional terms: how can other sectors, such as transport, education or taxation, improve health? The limitation of such an appeal is obvious because it is unclear why other sectors should invest resources or change what they are doing to improve health outcomes (Lynch, 2020). Transport, education and finance ministers often have other goals of more importance, and more accountability for outcomes other than health. Short of a total mobilization of government for health – something like the COVID-19 responses of 2020 in Europe – we should expect resistance from all sorts of interests to HiAP. That is exactly what HiAP researchers and practitioners found, for all that a large literature catalogued cases and examples of intersectoral action for health (Bacigalupe et al., 2010; Bekker et al., 2017; Greszczuk, 2019; Kickbusch, 2010; Koivusalo, 2010; Leppo et al., 2013; De Leeuw, 2022; McQueen et al., 2012; Marmot et al., 2012; Ståhl et al., 2006). If there were not a large, well-timed and sustained political push for HiAP, the effort was likely to founder.

Or was it? While much HiAP literature is produced in and for health policy circles, and therefore emphasizes the impact of its policies on health, a quick look at the actual literature suggests that writers and practitioners alike were actually seeking win-win solutions. Rather than simply asking schools to feed children better quality food, they were highlighting the educational benefits of improved nutrition (Behrman, 1996; Maluccio et al., 2009). Rather than simply asking municipal governments to encourage active transportation through changes to the built environment, such as bike lanes and wider pavements, they also highlighted the benefits to cities' merchants, nightlife, and tourist appeal (Mueller et al., 2015; Poirier, 2018).

In other words, successful HiAP might be half of a win-win solution, in which better and more sustainable cities or better test scores for children come *with* rather than at the expense of health. It stands to reason, because the causal links connecting good health and reduced health inequalities with better overall and more equal outcomes in many arenas are well rehearsed (Greer et al., 2022b). It also stands to reason because health care systems can be such large actors, with strong independent effects on their societies, as employers, owners of large-scale infrastructure, high-technology industries and purchasers of goods and services. Finally, it stands to reason that the successes were not purely HiAP because the space that HiAP seems to leave for its advocates is simply so cramped and small; the amount of policy change associated with HiAP goes beyond what we should expect if it were really just about inducing well-established and powerful organizations to change their priorities on the basis of some persuasive arguments alone. Once we start to look for win-win solutions in HiAP, there are many to be found.

We call these win-win solutions the *logic of co-benefits*. Co-benefits occur when two or more goals result from the same policy. Rather than a zero-sum model of policy, in which resources and political attention are finite and a gain for health is a loss for another sector, the logic of co-benefits directs our attention to the areas in which a gain for health and health systems is a gain for other goals as well. Thinking this way opens up new political vistas: of political strategies, of governance mechanisms, of whole-of-government and whole-of-society coalitions of many different actors who can benefit from a policy or goal. It also brings the health politics literature more in line with the broad approach of political scientists, who emphasize coalitions of different interests and appeals to broad swathes of the public as part of the formula for political and policy success.

In this book, the basic question we are asking is: how do we develop collaboration between sectors to achieve goals that cannot be attained through better health and health policies? Put differently, how can we better understand and communicate the health effects and co-benefits that intersectoral action can produce? The book draws on and makes a case for changing the argument about intersectoral action, from one focusing on health and the health sector as the main beneficiary to one based on co-benefits, focusing on benefits for all sectors. It makes the case for a Health *for* All Policies approach that focuses on co-benefits between sectors.

This book uses the Sustainable Development Goals as the framework for identifying goals across sectors. The next section introduces and discusses the SDGs. The SDGs are a set of global goals, broken down into specific targets and indicators to monitor. SDG3, "Good health and wellbeing", is well known in global health circles. Its goals and the policies needed to attain them have long been discussed, enacted and evaluated. But a moment's reflection on the other sixteen SDGs highlights the extent to which health and health policies can contribute to their attainment.

It first frames the topic in terms of two causal axes (Greer et al., 2022b). One is the impact of improved health status on other SDGs – for example, better health can lead to better educational and employment results. This is ground often trodden by economists and other quantitative researchers, though qualitative research on the relationship between health and social behaviour is vast and informative. It is the area in which we focus on findings such as the destructive relationship between HIV status and employment (Levinsohn et al., 2013). The other is the impact of health systems and policies on other sectors. The health sector is a major employer, driver of economic activity, and user of infrastructure; all of these can contribute to other goals, such as equal access to good jobs and economic development.

In terms of policies, we should not understate the impact of health policies and sectors through mechanisms other than improved health. Health in All Policies was, more often than not, a call to action for other sectors; Health *for* All Policies is both a call to improve health and a way to achieve goals beyond health. Furthermore, it calls for the health sector to do better in understanding and directing its impact on the world beyond the health care it provides. How can health sector expenditure, combined with attention to sustainable cities, contribute to urbanism; or, combined with industrial policy, contribute to economic development; or, combined with an appreciation of climate change, contribute to stopping and mitigating the harms of global heating?

1.2   Attaining the SDGs: the role of health sector co-benefits

If the world has shared goals, they are the Sustainable Development Goals (Fig. 1.1). The SDGs are seventeen objectives covering issues as different as eliminating poverty, access to clean water and sanitation,

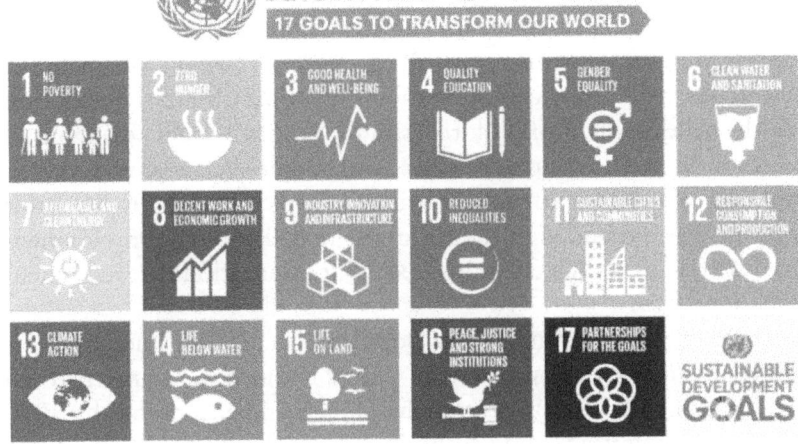

Fig. 1.1 The Sustainable Development Goals (SDGs) for 2027

and climate action, agreed upon by heads of government through the UN. They are not just the framework for UN action, but also receive at least some attention in government and other organizations' planning; for example, the European Union has replaced its Europe 2020 goals, in important mechanisms such as the European Semester, with the SDGs (Greer et al., 2022b). Even for those who are cynical about the actual adherence of governments to all seventeen goals, the SDGs provide a way to speak about widely held and important objectives. They are, in their intricacy, like a basket: while an individual strand might not be of interest, once woven together they encompass shared human goals.

The concept which became the Sustainable Development Goals is about as old as international law. Still, their core context is that of the UN and the international system as founded after the Second World War (Cueto, Brown & Fee, 2019). In 1948, Article 25 of the Universal Declaration of Human Rights stated that "everyone has the right to a standard of living adequate for the health and well-being of himself and of his family, including food, clothing, housing and medical care and necessary social services" (United Nations General Assembly, 1948). By the 1970s the idea of the right to health was developed further in the World Health Organization's (WHO) Health for All promotion, which envisioned securing the health and wellbeing of people worldwide. In combination, access to basic health services was affirmed as a fundamental human right in the Declaration of Alma Ata in 1978 (primary health care is key). Some goals included that at least 5% of the gross national product should be spent on health, at least 90% of children should have a weight for age that corresponds to the reference values, and people should have access to trained personnel for attending pregnancy and childbirth. In 2000, this concept was expanded in the form of the Millennium Development Goals (MDGs), which encompassed eight international development goals for 2015.

In 2015, the Sustainable Development Goals, also known as the Global Goals, were adopted by the United Nations as "a universal call to action to end poverty, protect the planet, and ensure that by 2030 all people enjoy peace and prosperity" (United Nations Development Programme, 2022). The 17 sectoral goals, see Fig. 1.1, come with numerous specific targets and indicators to propose suitable programmes to achieve the various goals. The SDGs are special insofar as they go further than many of their predecessor international policies. Health for All (HFA), the WHO health policy framework, for example, stressed the need for intersectorality but only defined targets for the health sector. The MDGs went further as they included targets on social development. In this respect, the SDGs can be seen as a consequential development as they literally comprise all policies and sectors. The SDGs are also very relevant as a platform for intersectoral programmes because they are more widely known than their predecessors and have been adopted by the entire UN System, the European Commission and many Member States.

Combining the notion of HiAP with this new set of goals, the idea is to recognize that an action in one sector can positively affect the outcome in other sectors. That said, if the goal is to advance wellbeing in our societies through strengthening the link with health, the SDGs can provide an excellent platform for intersectoral programmes. While the SDGs are not the only way to design intersectoral programmes, and the SDGs are not the only conceptual framework for human development, they are used here in this study as examples of how such programmes could be designed.

Box 1.2 How health care systems can help or hurt other SDGs: the case of a hospital

Health *for* All Policies means we need to look at ways that the health sector and health policies do or do not contribute to broader social goods. Imagine the development of a hospital, newly built, efficient, and located on the outskirts of the city, in an area primarily accessible by car. What is the hospital's impact on key policies highlighted in the SDGs? What could be done better if we were to seek co-benefits rather than simply the efficient production of health care services?

Climate action (SDG13) calls for a move to carbon neutrality while hospitals are a key source of greenhouse gas (GHG) emissions (Tennison et al., 2021). In the UK, the NHS is responsible for 4% of total national carbon emissions, of which 79% come from primary care and community services (NHS, 2012). Of these emissions, hospitals, which are large buildings requiring 24/7 energy for heating, ventilation, lighting and advanced energy-intensive medical devices and pharmaceuticals, are the greatest contributor (Eckelman & Sherman, 2016). NHS-related travel explains 3.5% of all road travel in the UK, making travel the 5th highest contributor of GHG emissions in the hospital system following medical equipment, pharmaceuticals, business services, fuels and electricity (NHS, 2012). The high use of energy in hospitals also creates an opportunity for hospitals to impact the SDG of accelerating renewable energy use (SDG7). Currently, most hospitals rely on non-renewable sources of energy. Studies have shown switching to renewable sources can contribute to sustainable development goals while also creating savings for hospitals (Prada et al., 2020; Sala, Alcamo & Nelli, 2016; Vaziri, Rezaee & Monirian, 2020).

In addition to energy, hospitals are large consumers of water impacting SDGs 6 and 12: Clean Water and Sanitation, and Responsible Consumption and Production, respectively. In 2017 the NHS utilized water equivalent to the total water use of Estonia (Sala, Alcamo & Nelli, 2016). In Spain, 900 hospitals account for 7% of the total use of water in the country, which amounts to roughly $600 million euros (Garcia-Sanz-Calcedo et al., 2017). The use of water in hospitals comes mostly from direct use (35–70%), research and treatment (15–40%) and food preparation (5–25%). Studies find this elevated water use could be limited with more responsible monitoring and auditing of water use (McGain & Naylor, 2014).

Hospital development can also impact SDGs of decent work (SDG8) and reduce inequality (SDG10). Hospitals are staff intensive and offer

Box 1.2 (cont.)

high opportunities for employment in the regions where they are located. In France, an average public hospital employs 876 people (Clark & Milcent, 2011). Locating these hospitals in suburban areas may provide employment opportunities in already prosperous areas, increasing employment inequity between suburban, urban and rural communities. In addition to employment inequality, hospitals and hospital location can increase inequality in health care access. Reliance on political will for funding and development of hospitals may lead to a lack of access to hospital care in marginalized communities (Matheson et al., 2018). Even when hospitals are accessed by these marginalized communities, poor hospital culture, such as embedded systematic racism, may lead to differences in treatment among groups (Matheson et al., 2018). Additionally, hospitals are generally resistant to change and show a lack of responsiveness to community needs, which has a greater impact on quality health care access in marginalized communities (Matheson et al., 2018).

Box 1.3 Why equity matters

There are two reasons why health equity is a necessary part of Health for All Policies.

The first is ethical: equity is a compelling value in its own right. Not only is it explicitly the purpose of some SDGs (5, gender equality, and 10, reduced inequalities), it is a goal spread throughout the other SDGs, whether that means the commitment to equal education in SDG4 or the commitment to good work and jobs for *all* in SDG8. Even if we disregard the SDGs, equity is a fundamental value of health and social policy, and policies that disregard equity are ethically problematic.

The second is simply that inequity can drag down a whole society. Unusually bad outcomes for a particular group that is victimized in some way – by racism, economic inequality, gender discrimination or similar mechanisms – will drag down the results for the whole country. The tails of the distribution affect the mean. The United States, for example, has the highest maternal mortality among rich countries. This is because of unusually high *Black* maternal mortality due to racism (Declercq & Zephyrin, 2020). The United States' overall bad outcome is not a result of processes that affect every person giving birth; it is a result of inequity, and addressing the overall bad outcome requires addressing the inequity.

Attaining the SDGs without attention to health equity is simply not possible.

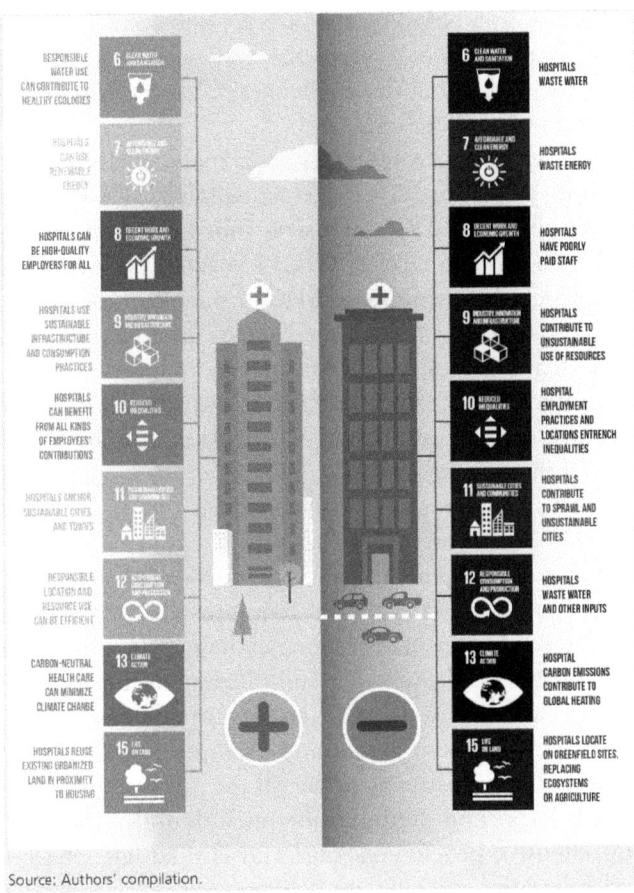

Source: Authors' compilation.

Fig. 1.2 Health care for all policies?

1.3 Summary of subsequent chapters

The book continues with Chapter 2 presenting the two causal chains that link health outcomes and health policies and organizations to other SDGs. We identify the methodological challenges of identifying and measuring co-benefits, discussing the quantitative, modelling and policy analysis approaches that can be used to forecast the effects of Health for All Policies approaches and then evaluate them. In Chapter 3, we address the weak spot of all intersectoral action: the political and governance challenges. It presents a framework for identifying promising areas for intersectoral action based on the salience and conflict associated with the issue, then identifies governance challenges and presents a set of techniques for addressing the challenges. Chapter 4 identifies some key lessons and policy directions.

Chapters 5–13 cover nine selected SDG cases including, SDG1 no poverty, SDG4 quality education, SDG5 gender equality, SDG8 decent work and economic growth, SDG9 industry, innovation and infrastructure, SDG10 reduced inequalities, SDG11 sustainable cities and communities, SDG13 climate action and SDG17 partnerships for the goals and their relationship to SDG3 health. Each of these chapters will showcase an in-depth analysis of the specific SDGs. In addition, country examples will depict the possibility of intersectoral collaboration between the SDG in question and SDG3 health using the analytical frameworks outlined in Chapters 2–4.

Chapter 5 discusses SDG Goal 1: "Ending poverty in all its forms everywhere". It argues that poorly designed coverage policies are a significant problem in the fight against poverty as they leave some of the sickest patients on the brink of financial ruin. To improve health coverage design, policies are needed to ensure that financially vulnerable people are not exposed to further hardship as a result of using health services. This chapter uses the cases of Latvia and Germany to demonstrate the relative importance of copayment design and exemptions in reducing poverty. Increasing public investment in health overall is a good first step; however, other important action points include full population coverage, a comprehensive benefits package and limited user charges to improve health outcomes and help eradicate poverty.

Chapter 6 looks at SDG4: quality education. Due to the fact that education is strongly associated with life expectancy, morbidity and health behaviours, it is widely recognized that health and education are mutually influential. While the focus has primarily been on the impact of education on health, advancing health and wellbeing remains a critical pathway to achieving education and lifelong learning. As such, a reorientation of systemic thinking and practice that builds on health and wellbeing as central elements of achieving quality education during the life course is key to achieving SDG4 quality education.

Chapter 7 argues that health care needs to include equity and access for women, men and all other genders. The reverse is also necessary: gender equality and human rights need health equity. This strong connection between SDG3 (health) and SDG5 (gender) creates specific conditions of co-benefits. However, bringing a gender lens to the debate over SDG co-benefits raises more general questions about universalist policy concepts, which assume "neutrality" and do not adequately respond to policy contexts and stakeholders' diverse needs and interests. This chapter ultimately calls for increased attention to gender equality and intersectionality, thereby capturing and addressing the importance of participatory governance more effectively. Two empirical case studies illustrate an optimum scenario of health action creating gender equality co-benefits with a focus on women's health.

Chapter 8 asserts that decent work and economic growth benefits greatly from a healthy population. In this vein, health policy itself can promote improved work and employment by making health sectors better employers. There are many opportunities to improve the quality of jobs and reduce inequalities, beginning with addressing particular management behaviours in particular units, to strong and well enforced anti-discrimination law, and paying a higher minimum wage. The political difficulty of making such adjustments, especially in the eyes of managers and policymakers, takes the form of added costs to organizations and reduced pay differentials that benefit higher-paid workers. The goal is thus to focus efforts on political actors such as unions and civil society that will support SDG8. A case study of Romania presents an overview of policy actions taken to address health workforce shortages, by tackling issues related to recruitment, retention and international mobility of health workers.

Chapter 9 points to the fact that initiatives such as technology transfer and local production of pharmaceuticals in low- and middle-income countries can be a means to promote industrial and innovation goals (SDG9), while meeting health needs. The main goal is to strengthen regulatory systems through local production. This will not only allow for the increased assessment of manufacturing practices and heightened quality control but will also provide additional opportunities to train and develop human resources, develop new skills, and promote local industrial development. The cases of Brazil and Mozambique illustrate the intersectoral initiatives between health and industrial policies and how they have ultimately led to increased health benefits.

The goal of Chapter 10 is to demonstrate how SDG3 (health for all) can work with SDG10 (reduce inequalities) to fight longstanding societal inequalities. One of the first steps is the creation of a National Health Insurance (NHI), whose goal is to cover the entire population with adequate health care at an affordable price. Health and health outcomes are, however, not only affected by the provision or access to health care and health services. They result from multidimensional and complex factors linked to the social determinants of health. So, while NHI may reduce inequality and inequity in health care, further attention will need to be placed on socioeconomic inequality given the social and economic disparities among the population groups in the country.

Chapter 11 argues that by using a multisectoral urban governance approach that emphasizes health, cities can expand successfully and equitably while leaving no residents behind. Two case studies will provide examples of interventions that have been implemented through a multisectoral approach, using urban planning strategies to impact health. As countries look to improve their commitment to building sustainable, healthy, inclusive and resilient cities (SDG11), stronger coordination across multiple sectors is needed to ensure policies and programmes targeting equitable growth are in place to prevent the negative consequences of rapid urbanization.

Chapter 12 shows how health systems and policy can address climate change. It uses the case study of the city of Toronto in Canada to offer lessons for directly involving health systems in subnational climate action as policy stakeholders and implementors, and the co-benefits health system engagement brings to promote climate action intersectorally. Health Systems as Stakeholders and Implementors in Climate Policy Change (SDG13) may take immediate steps through both: 1) participating in local planning for adverse weather events, and 2) making direct infrastructure investments in sustainable buildings and materials.

Chapter 13 examines the wide-ranging and often poorly understood SDG17 (Means of Implementation) in the context of health policy and governance. It fundamentally asks: How can health policies and systems contribute to achieving goals from SDG17? The author argues that there are significant synergies between health policy and SDG17 as many of the factors that potentially make "sustainable development" possible require healthy populations and functional health systems. When health and sustainable growth goals align, good population health, resting on environmentally sustainable food chains, adequate support for public health systems, good access to health care, and good enough governance for health, can provide benefits to the global economy and help to move towards a model of sustainable development.

1.4 Conclusion

Health for All Policies is a framework emphasizing co-benefits: the ways in which improved health or better health systems and policies can attain other goals. In terms of the SDGs, it captures the extent to which better health status, and use of health budgets, policies and infrastructures, can contribute to all of the SDGs, whether fairly obvious ones (health enables education) to ones that require more thought (health care systems' procurement and waste disposal systems affect life under the seas).

The case for co-benefits is not just that it shows what health policy can do for other goals. It is not just that it shows what health policy *should* do for other goals such as sustainability or reducing gender and other inequalities. It also opens up new perspectives on coalitions, politics and governance. It puts the focus on win-win solutions and the coalitions that can create them. Political and policy changes often happen when coalitions change, and one way to promote that is to identify new shared goals and agreements on policies.

This book is part of a broader package of work (Greer et al., 2022b), and focuses primarily on the ways in which health care *policies and systems* can produce co-benefits for other sectors, from reducing poverty (SDG1) to international partnership (SDG17). Other work in the package, drawing on the methods and literature discussed in Chapter 2, will focus on the co-benefits of improved health status. This book speaks to health care: one of the largest, most geographically distributed, technology-heavy, employment-heavy, education-focused and infrastructure-heavy sectors in the world. Health care purchasing, employment, research, training, estate, hiring and waste disposal decisions shape much of the world around us. What are the co-benefits of health systems and policies – and what can health policymakers do to make health policy for all policies?

References

Bacigalupe A, Esnaola S, Martin U et al. (2010). Learning lessons from past mistakes: how can Health in All Policies fulfill its promises? J Epidemiol Community Health, 64(6):504–505. (http://jech.bmj.com/content/64/6/504 .long)

Behrman JR (1996). The impact of health and nutrition on education. World Bank Res Obs, 11(1):23–37.

Bekker M, Helderman JK, Jansen M et al. (2017). The conditions and contributions of 'Whole of Society' governance in the Dutch 'All about Health ... ' programme. In: Greer SL, Wismar M, Pastorino G et al. (eds.) Civil society and health: Contributions and potential. Brussels: European Observatory on Health Systems and Policies; 159–180.

Chorev N (2012). The World Health Organization between North and South. Cornell University Press.

Clark AE, Milcent C (2011). Public employment and political pressure: the case of French hospitals. J Health Econ, 30(5):1103–1112. (https://doi .org/10.1016/j.jhealeco.2011.07.007)

Cueto M, Brown TM, Fee E (2019). The world health organization: A history. Cambridge University Press.

Cylus J, Permanand G, Smith PC (2018). Making the economic case for investing in health systems: What is the evidence that health systems advance economic and fiscal objectives.

Declercq E, Zephyrin L (2020). Maternal mortality in the United States: a primer. Commonwealth Fund.

De Leeuw E (2022). Intersectorality and health: a glossary. J Epidemiol Community Health, 76:206–208.

Eckelman MJ, Sherman J (2016). Environmental impacts of the U.S. health care system and effects on Public Health. PLOS ONE, 11(6). (https://doi .org/10.1371/journal.pone.0157014)

Fukuda-Parr S (2018). Sustainable development goals. In: Greer SL, Falkenbach M, Siciliani L et al. (eds). (2022). From Health in All Policies to Health for All Policies. The Lancet Public Health. (https://doi.org/10.1016/ S2468-2667(22)00155-4)

Garcia-Sanz-Calcedo J, Lopez-Rodriguez F, Yusaf T, Al-Kassir A (2017). Analysis of the average annual consumption of water in the hospitals of Extremadura (Spain). Energies, 10(4):479. (https://doi.org/10.3390/en10040479)

Greer SL, King EJ, da Fonseca EM et al. (eds). (2021). Coronavirus Politics: The Comparative Politics and Policy of COVID-19. Ann Arbor: University of Michigan Press.

Greer SL, Fonseca EM, Raj M, Willison C (2022a). Institutions and the politics of agency in COVID-19 response: Federalism, executive power, and public health policy in Brazil, India, and the US. J Soc Policy. doi:10.1017/ S0047279422000642.

Greer SL, Rozenblum S, Fahy N et al. (2022b). Everything you always wanted to know about European Union health policy but were afraid to ask (3rd, completely revised ed.). Brussels: WHO/European Observatory on Health Systems and Policies.

Greszczuk C (2019). Implementing health in all policies. Health Foundation. (https://www.health.org.uk/sites/default/files/upload/publications/2019/Implementing%20health%20in%20all%20policies.pdf)

Kickbusch I (2010). Health in all policies: the evolution of the concept of horizontal health governance. Implementing health in all policies: Adelaide; 11–24.

Koivusalo M (2010). The state of Health in All Policies (HiAP) in the European Union: potential and pitfalls. J Epidemiol Community Health, 64(6):500–503. doi:10.1136/jech.2009.102020.

Lawn JE, Rohde J, Rifkin S et al. (2008). Alma-Ata 30 years on: revolutionary, relevant, and time to revitalize. Lancet, 372(9642):917–927. doi:10.1016/S0140-6736(08)61402-6.

Leppo K, Ollila E, Peña S et al. (eds). (2013). Health in All Policies – Seizing opportunities, implementing policies. STM.

Levinsohn J, McLaren ZM, Shisana O et al. (2013). HIV Status and Labor Market Participation in South Africa. Rev Econ Stat, 95(1):98–108. doi:10.1162/REST_a_00237.

Lynch J (2020). Regimes of inequality: the political economy of health and wealth. Cambridge University Press.

McGain F, Naylor C (2014). Environmental sustainability in hospitals – A systematic review and Research Agenda. J Health Serv Res Policy, 19(4):245–252. (https://doi.org/10.1177/1355819614534836)

McQueen D, Wismar M, Lin V et al. (2012). Inter-sectoral governance for Health in All Policies: Structures, actions and experiences. Copenhagen: WHO Regional Office for Europe/European Observatory on Health Systems and Policies.

Maluccio JA et al. (2009). The impact of improving nutrition during early childhood on education among Guatemalan adults. Econ J, 119(537):734–763.

Marmot M, Allen J, Bell R et al. (2012). WHO European review of social determinants of health and the health divide. Lancet, 380(9846):1011–1029. doi:10.1016/S0140-6736(12)61228-8.

Matheson A et al. (2018). Lowering hospital walls to achieve health equity. BMJ. (https://doi.org/10.1136/bmj.k3597)

Mueller N et al. (2015). Health impact assessment of active transportation: a systematic review. Prev med, 76:103–114.

NHS (2012). The NHS: Carbon Footprint. NHS Public Health Special Interest Group – Sustainable Development.

Poirier JA (2018). Bicycle lanes and business success: A San Francisco examination. Transp Res Rec, 2672(7):47–57.

Prada M et al. (2020). New solutions to reduce greenhouse gas emissions through energy efficiency of buildings of special importance – hospitals. Sci Total Environ, 718:137446. (https://doi.org/10.1016/j.scitotenv.2020.137446)

Sagan A, Webb E, Azzopardi-Muscat N et al. (2021). Health systems resilience during covid-19. Lessons for building back better. United Kingdom: World Health Organization, European Commission, European Observatory on Health Systems and Policies.

Sala M, Alcamo G, Nelli LC (2016). Energy-saving solutions for five hospitals in Europe. Mediterranean Green Buildings & Renewable Energy, 1–17. doi:https://doi.org/10.1007/978-3-319-30746-6_1.

Ståhl T, Wismar M, Ollila E et al. (eds). (2006). Health in all policies: prospects and potentials. Finland: Ministry of Social Affairs and Health.

Tennison I et al. (2021). Health care's response to climate change: a carbon footprint assessment of the NHS in England. Lancet Planet Health, 5(2):e84–e92.

United Nations Development Programme (2022). The SDGs in Action. (https://www.undp.org/sustainable-development-goals, 10 February 2022)

United Nations General Assembly (1948). Universal Declaration of Human Rights (Article 25). Paris, France. (https://www.un.org/en/about-us/universal-declaration-of-human-rights, 10 February 2022)

Vaziri SM, Rezaee B, Monirian MA (2020). Utilizing renewable energy sources efficiently in hospitals using demand dispatch. Renew Energy, 151:551–62.

Weber M (2020). From Alma Ata to the SDGs: The Politics of Global Health Governance and the Elusive "Health for All". Global Governance: A Review of Multilateralism and International Organizations, 26(1):176–197.

WHO (2014). Health in all policies: Helsinki statement. Framework for country action. World Health Organization.

2 | *Finding and understanding co-benefits*

SCOTT L. GREER, MICHELLE FALKENBACH,
LUIGI SICILIANI, JANAMARIE PERROUD,
MARIE CHANTEL MONTÁS, MATTHIAS WISMAR

2.1 Introduction

HiAP and "healthy public policies are well known uses" of the basic intuition behind co-benefits, but there are others. The Healthy Cities movement, for example, focused on the ways in which urban functions not always understood as being about health could contribute to better health and, therefore, better cities (Ashton, 2002; De Leeuw, 2001; De Leeuw et al., 2015).

Each of these, and other policy agendas, focused on how policies intended to do something other than improve health and how improved health and policies can contribute to another agenda. A focus on wins for the health sector, though, has the obvious drawback that people with primary goals other than health might not be interested – because their economic, political, career or other incentives and interests lead them to focus on other issues. Decades of "new public management", for example, have explicitly tried to focus different parts of the public sector on a small number of specific goals, such as test results for schools and waiting times for health care systems. It is hard to undo such accountability systems and tell schools that they are also expected to improve student health and hospitals that they should be better employers (Box 2.1).

We propose to go beyond Health *in* All Policies to focus on Health *for* All Policies (Fig. 2.1). Health *for* All Policies is focused on *co-benefits*, policy outcomes that affect all involved sectors positively regardless of which sector provides the policy outputs (Greer et al., 2022). In this, we build on a trend in HiAP literature to focus on win-win solutions between sectors: not asking policymakers in transport, education or agriculture to solve health problems, but focusing on ways that health outcomes and policies can create win-win solutions. We can see this shift in newer work which stresses that policy should be built on the "principle of co-benefits: all parties that contribute should benefit

Box 2.1 Analysing the impact of health on other SDGs

In health systems, we want to produce policy changes that ultimately improve outcomes and equity while reducing disparities in population health. Econometrics and statistical models can be used as a tool to create robust frameworks to estimate the impact of better health on other social outcomes (Abadie & Cattaneo, 2018; Angrist & Pischke, 2008, 2015; Cunningham, 2021; Gertler et al., 2010).

Experimental designs with phased-in randomized control trials (RCTs) are a gold standard for analysing the impact of health technologies and drugs, but these are too costly or often unfeasible when it comes to evaluating the effect of programmes and policies and their influence on earning, labour, productivity, and educational attainment, among others (Dillon, Friedman & Serneels, 2021; Miguel & Kremer, 2004). However, RCTs are not the most popular in this field due to the time and resource investment they entail. Quasi-experimental methods, including difference-in-difference (DiD) estimators, regression discontinuity designs, instrumental variables, matching techniques and other robust multivariate regressions, dominate the econometrics field for causal inference (Angrist & Pischke, 2010; Dimick & Ryan, 2014). For instance, to measure different health shocks in Denmark and their effect on labour supply, authors create a DiD to look at households that experienced strokes and heart attacks, identifying the treatment effect, and constructing counterfactuals to affected households (Fadlon & Nielsen, 2021).

Econometric models can quantify the effect of a health or health policy or programme on other outcomes (Imbens & Wooldridge, 2009). This is crucial to support the development of Health for all policies and achieve cross-sectoral involvement between actors.

Sources:

Abadie A, Cattaneo MD (2018). Econometric Methods for Program Evaluation. *Annual Review of Economics*, 10(1):465–503. (https://doi.org/10.1146/annurev-economics-080217-053402)

Angrist JD, Pischke J-S (2008). *Mostly harmless econometrics: An empiricist's companion*. Princeton University Press.

Angrist JD, Pischke J-S (2010). The Credibility Revolution in Empirical Economics: How Better Research Design is Taking the Con out of Econometrics. *J Econ Perspectives*, 24(2):3–30. (https://doi.org/10.1257/jep.24.2.3)

Angrist JD, Pischke J-S (2015). *Mastering 'metrics: The path from cause to effect*. Princeton University Press.

Box 2.1 (cont.)

Cunningham S (2021). Inference. In *Cunningham S. Causal Inference: The Mixtape*. Yale University Press; 423–424.

Dillon A, Friedman J, Serneels P (2021). Health Information, Treatment, and Worker Productivity. *J Eur Econ Assoc*, 19(2):1077–1115. https://doi.org/10.1093/jeea/jvaa024

Dimick JB, Ryan AM (2014). Methods for Evaluating Changes in Health Care Policy: The Difference-in-Differences Approach. *JAMA*, 312(22):2401. (https://doi.org/10.1001/jama.2014.16153)

Fadlon I, Nielsen TH (2021). Family Labor Supply Responses to Severe Health Shocks: Evidence from Danish Administrative Records. *Am Econ J: Appl Econ*, 13(3):1–30. (https://doi.org/10.1257/app.20170604)

Gertler P, Martinez S, Premand P et al. (2010). *Impact Evaluation in Practice*. World Bank Publications.

Imbens GW, Wooldridge JM (2009). Recent Developments in the Econometrics of Program Evaluation. *J Econ Lit*, 47(1):5–86. (https://doi.org/10.1257/jel.47.1.5)

Impact Evaluation in Practice, Second Edition (world). (n.d.). Stand Alone Books. (https://elibrary.worldbank.org/doi/pdf/10.1596/978-1-4648-0779-4, 28 September 2022)

Miguel E, Kremer M (2004). Worms: Identifying Impacts on Education and Health in the Presence of Treatment Externalities. *Econometrica*, 72(1):159–217. (https://doi.org/10.1111/j.1468-0262.2004.00481.x)

from being involved. As well as improving health and health equity, partnerships should support other sectors to achieve their own goals, such as creating good-quality jobs or local economic stability. At the same time, a healthier population is likely to bring social and economic benefits to other sectors in the long term. This offers further rationale for cross-sectoral investment" (Greszczuk, 2019).

Co-benefits are benefits of a policy in multiple sectors: ways in which a single policy (for example, reduction of inequalities in child health) leads to a variety of beneficial outcomes (for example, reduction of inequalities in educational performance, employment outcomes and political participation). They are win-win policies which achieve goals across multiple policy sectors and, politically, help to transcend the sectoral logic of much policymaking. Health *for* All Policies captures a wider range of interactions (Fig. 2.1).

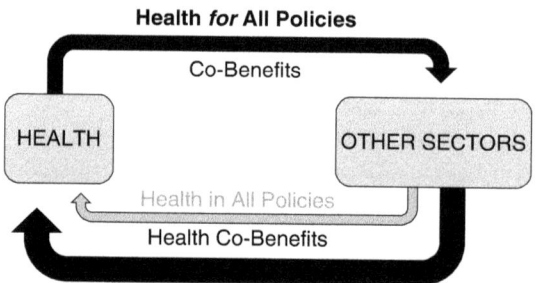

Fig. 2.1 Causal connections in Health for All Policies

There are many examples of co-benefits in practice and research literature because many kinds of policies have intended or unintended effects beyond their main targets. Reducing catastrophic health care costs can be a goal of health care coverage policy; poverty reduction is a co-benefit. Building a hospital with good walking, cycling and public transport connections can have co-benefits for cities and the climate. Greater equity in health care can help reduce a variety of disparities in the workplace.

The logic of co-benefits focuses our attention on identifying and removing problems, such as negative externalities or co-disbenefits, and identifying win-win rather than win-lose intersectoral solutions. The complexity of public policy encourages such a focus on win-win solutions because there are usually degrees of freedom in every step of policy formulation and implementation, which allow the creation of positive-sum relationships instead of tradeoffs. Without denying the existence of tradeoffs and zero- or negative-sum policy conflicts, we can still emphasize thinking about policymaking in ways that reduce their extent.

There are two compelling reasons to consider policies in a Health for All Policies framework. The first, the subject of the rest of this chapter, is that it allows us to do more with less. COVID-19 came against the backdrop of decades of austerity and recalibration, rather than growth, in social and health policy expenditure. Pandemic response was a fiscal policy challenge for many governments, and even those that mustered the resources for a successful social policy response are likely to be having debates about retrenchment and priorities. Investments in health are more likely to be palatable if they can be shown to produce benefits outside the health sector, just as investments in other sectors might become more attractive if they produce health.

Using this logic, we can gain more value from our health policies and investments. Health care is an immense area of public expenditure, and one with a large physical infrastructure, workforce at all levels of qualifications and income, extensive science and research base, strong impact on mobility patterns, and large consumption of goods from potatoes to very high technology instruments. Purchasing, employment, locational and other decisions in the health sector are often made without much systematic regard for their effects on broader policy areas. Support for health care investment – and actual ability to achieve other goals – would be higher if policymakers tapped the potential impact of health care decisionmaking on broader policies. Public health interventions, likewise, are often framed purely in terms of aggregate health status or equity effects, but the economic, social and environmental consequences should be part of their justification. The COVID-19 pandemic, in good and bad ways, showed the need to understand the impact of public health measures and their effects on other goals such as education, unemployment and social services (Greer et al., 2021; Sagan et al., 2021).

The second reason is that it allows us to build new and stronger political coalitions. One of the problems of Health in All Policies is that it could look like health ministers trying to divert other departments' resources at the expense of their own obligations, priorities, politics, skills and accountability relationships. Its focus on benefits to the health sector can imply a negative-sum relationship between sectors, one that is visible in government budgeting practices that clarify how money spent on health is not being spent on anything else. By contrast, a focus on co-benefits is a search for win-win solutions: ways that other sectors can benefit from health policy and investment, and ways that health policy and investment can produce benefits for other sectors.

2.2 The two routes to co-benefits

There are two ways in which health policy can contribute to achieving other goals, i.e., co-benefits (see Fig. 2.2). The first is through the *contribution of health status to other outcomes*, or the way in which improved health status and reduced health inequalities contribute to goals outside the health domain. On this route, better and more equal

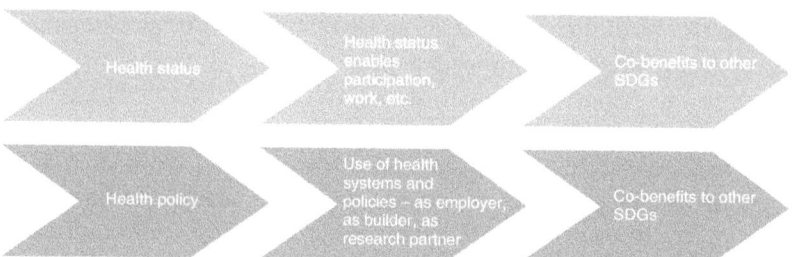

Fig. 2.2 Two causal pathways

population health contributes to the attainment of other goals. For example, the health of children influences their educational attainment (SDG4), and health inequities influence the ability of women (SDG5), the poor, and vulnerable groups (SDG10) to receive the benefits of education and then secure equal access to good jobs (SDG8). Health status even influences political participation and civil society engagement (SDG16), and ill health can cause catastrophic health care payments that can make people fall into poverty (SDG1).

The second way health policy can contribute to achieving other goals, i.e., co-benefits, is through the *contribution of health policy to other outcomes*, or co-benefits coming from health policies. This route alludes to specific health policy interventions that contribute to goals outside the health domain. Health policies and systems are big economic and social actors that affect their societies. Their behaviour as employers can shape labour markets. Their decisions about buildings and design can affect urban life and environmental sustainability. The extent of financial protection that they afford to their users can affect poverty and inequality (Thomson et al., 2020).

If we consider this first route, the contribution of health status to other SDGs, we find that there is an extensive existing literature to build upon (Haines, 2017; Howden-Chapman & Chapman, 2012; Jack & Kinney, 2010; Sharifi et al., 2021; Shaw et al., 2014). In relation to education (SDG4), Alam (2015) shows, using longitudinal data and panel-data methods, that in Tanzania, a father's illness decreases children's school attendance by 5% and decreases children's likelihood of completing primary school by 25%, leading to one and a half fewer years of schooling. Concerning employment (SDG8), Dillon, Friedman and Serneels (2021) use a phased-in randomized design, showing that preventing malaria infection in Nigeria can increase earnings by about 10%. Fadlon and Nielsen (2021) show, using differences-in-differences and matching methods, that severe non-fatal health shocks such as a heart attack or stroke in Denmark reduce earnings by 18% and household income by 3.4%; in contrast, fatal health shocks lead to increases in surviving spouses' labour force participation by 7.5% and annual labour income by 6.8%. Jockers et al. (2021), using an instrumental variable method, show that large-scale HIV antiretroviral therapy programmes in South Africa improve life expectancy and reduce absenteeism rates among workers living with HIV by about twelve days per year. Eriksen and colleagues, using differences-in-differences methods, show that the onset of type 1 diabetes in children induces mothers to shift to part-time work and experience a long-term 4–5% decrease in wage income in Denmark (Eriksen et al., 2021). For political participation (SDG16), Constantino, Cooperman and Moreira (2021) show that higher COVID-19 incidence near the time of the election in Brazil is associated with lower voter turnout. These various pieces of literature can inform how health status affects other aspects of life by estimating the likely effect of improvements in health status on other goals.

Researchers have made great progress in developing quantitative methods that can inform policy. Box 2.1 and 2.2 show two useful approaches, discussed in more detail in Greer et al. (2022). Box 2.1 focuses on quantitative empirical approaches, showing how they can develop firm quantitative evidence about the impact of health status and outcomes on other policy areas. Box 2.2 shows how modelling can then allow policymakers to anticipate the impact of improved health on other areas.

Box 2.2 Harnessing models for Health for All Policies

Mathematical models use theoretical frameworks and equations to relate components of a system to each other (Panovska-Griffiths et al., 2021; Vanagas et al., 2019). In practice, these models can support the development of Health for All Policies by conceptualizing systems and how they will react to policies.

An understanding of the relationships between health and other sectors in a given context is critical in taking a Health for All Policies approach. System dynamics modelling can be useful in mapping these

Box 2.2 (cont.)

relationships. System dynamics is a complex systems approach to modelling that can be used to both identify *which parts* of the system interact, and characterize *how* they interact through feedback loops, delays and non-linear effects (Darabi & Hosseinichimeh, 2020). Moreover, system dynamics models can serve in a diagnostic capacity: identifying which modelled parameters and structures require change in order to achieve a desired outcome (Homer & Hirsch, 2006).

These models are particularly well suited to a Health *for* All Policies approach as they are not bound by directionality in their representations of relationships. While most system dynamics applications have used a Health *in* All Policies frame (Homer & Hirsch, 2006), extending the scope of these models to capture broader dynamics can expand the existing complex systems' perspective to health policy (Adam & de Savigny, 2012; Peters, 2014) and help inform the development of policies that produce co-benefits.

Models can also quantify co-benefits of health policies through the application of decision analyses. These methods employ decision models which provide a structural framework capable of synthesizing available data from a range of fields and evaluate outcomes of policy alternatives (Briggs et al., 2006; Kuntz et al., 2016). The specific models utilized will depend on the policy context and question at hand. They can include decision trees, Markov models and agent-based models. A key advantage of using decision models to estimate policy outcomes is their ability to handle data poor contexts and uncertainty (Kuntz et al., 2016). Decision models not only provide a structural framework for synthesizing data from disparate sources, but also allow for extrapolations that are often required to reflect the decision context appropriately.

Among decision analytic methods, Cost-Benefit Analysis (CBA) is particularly conducive to measuring co-benefits. Given that CBA measures all outcomes in monetary terms, it facilitates the inclusion of costs and effects beyond the domain of health (Owens et al., 2016). While the traditional application of CBA prioritizes efficiency over co-benefits, disaggregation among the costs and benefits allows for the identification and quantification of *win-win* outcomes characteristic of a co-benefiting policy. CBA has often been employed to evaluate impacts at the intersection of environmental and health policy (OECD, 2018), a practice that can be built upon with the Health for All Policies approach.

Box 2.2 (cont.)

Sources:

Adam T, de Savigny D (2012). Systems thinking for strengthening health systems in LMICs: need for a paradigm shift. *Health Policy Plan*, 27(suppl_4):iv1–iv3. (https://doi.org/10.1093/heapol/czs084)

Briggs AH, Claxton K, Sculpher MJ (2006). Decision Modelling for Health Economic Evaluation. Oxford University Press. (https://books.google.com/books?id=-vUJAQAAMAAJ)

Darabi N, Hosseinichimeh N (2020). System dynamics modeling in health and medicine: a systematic literature review. *Syst Dyn Rev*, 36(1):29–73. (https://doi.org/https://doi.org/10.1002/sdr.1646)

Homer JB, Hirsch GB (2006). System dynamics modeling for public health: background and opportunities. Am J Public Health, 96(3):452–458. (https://doi.org/10.2105/AJPH.2005.062059)

Kuntz KM, Russell LB, Owens DK et al. (2016). Decision Models in Cost-Effectiveness Analysis. In: Neumann PJ, Ganiats TG, Russell LB et al. (eds) Cost-Effectiveness in Health and Medicine. Oxford University Press; 105–136. (https://doi.org/10.1093/acprof:oso/9780190492939.001.0001)

OECD (2018). Cost-Benefit Analysis and the Environment. https://www.oecd.org/env/tools-evaluation/CBA-brochure-web.pdf

Owens DK, Siegel JE, Sculpher MJ et al. (2016). Designing a Cost-Effectiveness Analysis. In: Neumann PJ, Ganiats TG, Russell LB et al. (eds) Cost-Effectiveness in Health and Medicine. Oxford University Press; 75–104. (https://doi.org/10.1093/acprof:oso/9780190492939.001.0001)

Panovska-Griffiths J, Kerr C, Waites W et al. (2021). Mathematical modeling as a tool for policy decision making: Applications to the COVID-19 pandemic. Handb Stat, 44:291–326. (https://doi.org/10.1016/bs.host.2020.12.001)

Peters DH (2014). The application of systems thinking in health: why use systems thinking? Health Res Policy Syst, 12:51. (https://doi.org/10.1186/1478-4505-12-51)

Vanagas G, Krilavičius T, Man KL (2019). Mathematical Modeling and Models for Optimal Decision-Making in Health Care. Comput Math Methods Med, 2019:2945021–2945021. (https://doi.org/10.1155/2019/2945021)

2.3   Identifying co-benefits of health systems and policies

The core of this book is a focus on the second causal pathway, the one linking health systems and policies to other SDGs. How can the many decisions taken in the health sector, from infrastructure to hiring to purchasing, produce co-benefits that will work to the maximal benefit of citizens?

Identifying and estimating co-benefits from health systems and policies presents different methodological challenges. It is more dependent on sector-specific knowledge of causal mechanisms as well as contextual factors such as budgeting procedures, urban design or labour law, as seen in Box 2.3. Chapters 5–13 are chosen to illustrate the different ways we can understand the impact of health systems and policies, show the importance of policy expertise. It is difficult to "green the hospital" or turn health care expenditure into industrial development without a deep and interdisciplinary understanding of how the systems work. Expertise, and more often than not qualitative research, is necessary to understand the complexities of issues such as employment discrimination, infrastructure sustainability, and purchasing. That expertise and research can then be used, as we show in the chapters of this book, to identify the research approaches that can convincingly specify the relationships, identify the best approaches, and quantify the results.

Box 2.3 Understanding the impact of health systems and policies

How can we understand the impact of a given health policy on other SDGs, given the multiple causal pathways extending from hospital procurement to sustainability or health research policies to innovation?

It is possible to identify co-benefits in three steps. The goal is to build a logic model that can be used to argue for policies with co-benefits. The first is to understand basic relationships between the health care system and policies and the issue in question. This need not be hard: there is an obvious connection between the location and development of health care infrastructure and the sustainability, equity and attractiveness of the surrounding neighbourhoods. Health care systems' connection with good work and employment, or many aspects of equity, come through their role as employers.

The second step is to develop a logic model of the way policies can influence those relationships. For example, how can decisions about

---

Box 2.3 (cont.)

building a hospital (Box 1.2) influence different goals such as equitable employment and reducing carbon emissions? This asks for knowledge of the policy sector in the country context as well as the broader international literature on the relationships involved. The quality and extent of the international scholarly literature varies greatly from topic to topic, but it can map out basic mechanisms as well as some estimates from possibly relevant contexts. A policy model can also enable commissioning rapid research on particular topics in a particular context if necessary.

The third step is to identify the policies or actions with significant potential co-benefits and the most realistic chances of success and implementation. This means two things. It means trying to develop quantitative estimates of the benefits of a given policy. This quantitative research comes fairly far along in the process because it depends on a competent model of the relationship between the variables and a good understanding of how they can be convincingly specified. It means further analysis of the organizational requirements and barriers to implementation combined with an analysis of the potential coalition of supporters. This latter is very likely to involve qualitative research.

Box 2.3 presents an abstracted version of the approach, from which policies can be modelled. The box focuses on developing an understanding of the relationships, most often through an interdisciplinary approach that might require qualitative research. It is a conceptual presentation of the approach used in the case study chapters (Chapters 5–13) in this book, and could be used for other policy areas.

2.4 Identifying co-benefits of health status

If we consider the second route, the contribution of health policies to other outcomes outside the health domain, co-benefits have also been documented in the empirical evidence. For example, with poverty (SDG1), using differences-in-differences methods Limwattananon and colleagues show that a reform which greatly extended health insurance coverage in Thailand reduced out-of-pocket expenditure by 28% and reduced catastrophic payments by two percentage points (Limwattananon et al., 2015). Using a regression-discontinuity design approach, Bauhoff, Hotchkiss and Smith (2011) suggest that the Medical Insurance Programme for the Poor in the republic of Georgia decreased mean out-of-pocket expenditures for some groups and reduced the risk of high inpatient expenditures, though the programme did not affect the utilization of health services. In contrast, Bernal, Carpio and Klein (2017), using a regression discontinuity design, show that an expansion of health insurance coverage in Peru had large effects on measures of curative care use (individuals were more likely to visit a doctor by nine percentage points, to receive medicines by 15 percentage points, that a medical analysis is performed by five percentage points, to visit a hospital or receive surgery by eight percentage points) but increased out-of-pocket spending by 282 Soles, equivalent to 1.5% of household income, due to higher consumption of medicines, hospital visits and/ or surgeries not covered by insurance financed by households due to more awareness of health need. Hu and colleagues, using synthetic control methods, show that the Medicaid expansions under the 2010 Patient Protection and Affordable Care Act in the United States reduced the number of unpaid bills and the amount of debt sent to third-party collection agencies (Hu et al., 2018).

In relation to employment (SDG8), using differences-in-differences methods, Del Valle (2021) shows that the expansion of health insurance coverage in Mexico increased labour supply by reducing the likelihood of informal workers exiting the labour market by 15%. Goodman-Bacon (2021), using differences-in-differences methods, shows that children covered by Medicaid in the United States have a higher labour supply by four percentage points. Jeon and Pohl (2019), using matching methods, show that innovations in cancer treatment in Canada during the 1990s and 2000s reduced the negative employment effects of cancer by 63% to 70%. Beuermann and Pecha (2020), using differences-in-differences methods and a regression discontinuity design, show that the elimination of user fees in public health facilities in Jamaica reduced the number of sick days by 44% for individuals who were 40 to 64 years old.

For education (SDG4), Araújo and colleagues provide evidence that a large-scale iodine supplementation programme in Tanzania increased completed years of education and income scores in adulthood (Araújo, Carrillo & Sampaio, 2021). Bütikofer and Salvanes (2020), using differences-in-differences methods, show that cohorts of children subject to a tuberculosis control programme in Norway introduced in 1948 reduced missing school days by 9% in the short term and increased years of education by 0.5 years in the long term and earnings by 7%. Baranov and Kohler (2018), using differences-in-differences methods, show that access to antiretroviral therapy for AIDS in Malawi increases expenditures on education and children's schooling, and increases savings. Ozier (2018), using a phased randomized intervention design, shows that deworming interventions in Kenya had cognitive effects for children, which are equivalent to at least half a year of additional schooling. Brown and colleagues show that greater childhood Medicaid eligibility expansion in the United States increases college enrolment (Brown, Kowalski & Lurie, 2020). Bütikofer, Mølland and Salvanes (2018) show that the rollout of a free nutritious breakfast programme in schools in Norway increases education by 0.1 years and earnings by 2–3%.

2.5 Conclusion

The logic of co-benefits produces many theoretically interesting ideas, but to become convincing, it must be paired with competent policy analysis and evaluation. This will not always be easy, because developing methods can involve understanding complicated causal linkages between fields such as health care, urbanism, ecology and trade. But developing methods for scholarly and applied, practical government can be extremely important: how can budgeters, policy evaluators and other experts within and around government judge the plausibility of a co-benefits argument? How can their evaluative methods, so often seemingly dry and technical, support the identification and evaluation of co-benefits policies?

References

Alam SA (2015). Parental health shocks, child labor and educational outcomes: Evidence from Tanzania. J Health Econ, 44:161–175.

Araújo D, Carrillo B, Sampaio B (2021). The long-run economic consequences of iodine supplementation. J Health Econ, 79:102490.

Ashton JR (2002). Healthy cities and healthy settings. Promot Educ, 9(1_ suppl):12–14.

Baranov V, Kohler H-P (2018). The impact of AIDS treatment on savings and human capital investment in Malawi. Am Econ J Appl Econ, 10(1):266–306.

Bauhoff S, Hotchkiss DR, Smith O (2011). The impact of medical insurance for the poor in Georgia: a regression discontinuity approach. Health Econ, 20(11):1362–1378.

Bernal N, Carpio MA, Klein TJ (2017). The effects of access to health insurance: evidence from a regression discontinuity design in Peru. J Public Econ, 154:122–136.

Beuermann DW, Camilo JP (2020). The effects of weather shocks on early childhood development: Evidence from 25 years of tropical storms in Jamaica. Econ Hum Biol, 37: 100851.

Brown DW, Kowalski AE, Lurie IZ (2020). Long-term impacts of childhood Medicaid expansions on outcomes in adulthood. Rev Econ Stud, 87(2):792–821.

Bütikofer A, Salvanes KG (2020). Disease control and inequality reduction: Evidence from a tuberculosis testing and vaccination campaign. Rev Econ Stud, 87(5):2087–2125.

Bütikofer A, Mølland E, Salvanes KG (2018). Childhood nutrition and labor market outcomes: Evidence from a school breakfast program. J Public Econ, 168:62–80.

Constantino SM, Cooperman AD, Moreira TMQ (2021). Voting in a global pandemic: Assessing dueling influences of Covid-19 on turnout. Soc Sci Q, 102(5):2210–2235. doi:10.1111/ssqu.13038.

De Leeuw E (2001). Global and local (glocal) health: the WHO healthy cities programme. Global Change and Human Health, 2(1):34–45.

De Leeuw E, Kickbusch I, Palmer N et al. (2015). European Healthy Cities come to terms with health network governance. Health Promot Int, 30(suppl_1):i32–i44.

Del Valle A (2021). The effects of public health insurance in labor markets with informal jobs: Evidence from Mexico. J Health Econ, 77:102454.

Dillon A, Friedman J, Serneels P (2021). Health information, treatment, and worker productivity. J Eur Econ Assoc, 19(2):1077–1115.

Eriksen TLM, Gaulke A, Skipper N et al. (2021). The impact of childhood health shocks on parental labor supply. J Health Econ, 78:102486.

Fadlon I, Nielsen TH (2021). Family labor supply responses to severe health shocks: Evidence from Danish administrative records. Am Econ J Appl Econ, 13(3):1–30.

Goodman-Bacon A (2021). The long-run effects of childhood insurance coverage: Medicaid implementation, adult health, and labor market outcomes. Am Econ Rev, 111(8):2550–2593.

Greer SL, Jarman H, Falkenbach M et al. (2021). Social policy as an integral component of pandemic response: Learning from COVID-19 in Brazil, Germany, India and the United States. Glob Public Health, 16(8–9):1209–1222.

Greer SL, Falkenbach M, Siciliani L et al. (2022). From Health in All Policies to Health for All Policies. The Lancet Public Health. (https://doi.org/10.1016/S2468-2667(22)00155-4)

Greszczuk C (2019). Implementing health in all policies. Health Foundation. (https://www.health.org.uk/sites/default/files/upload/publications/2019/Implementing%20health%20in%20all%20policies.pdf)

Haines A (2017). Health co-benefits of climate action. Lancet Planetary Health 1(1):e4–e5.

Howden-Chapman P, Chapman R (2012). Health co-benefits from housing-related policies. Curr Opin Environ Sustain 4(4):414–419.

Hu L, Kaestner R, Mazumder B et al. (2018). The effect of the affordable care act Medicaid expansions on financial wellbeing. J Public Econ, 163:99–112.

Jack DW, Kinney PL (2010). Health co-benefits of climate mitigation in urban areas. Curr Opin Environ Sustain 2(3):172–177.

Jeon S-H, Pohl RV (2019). Medical innovation, education, and labor market outcomes of cancer patients. J Health Econ, 68:102228.

Jockers D, Langlotz S, French D et al. (2021). HIV treatment and worker absenteeism: Quasi-experimental evidence from a large-scale health program in South Africa. J Health Econ, 79:102479.

Limwattananon S, Neelsen S, O'Donnell O et al. (2015). Universal coverage with supply-side reform: The impact on medical expenditure risk and utilization in Thailand. J Public Econ, 121:79–94.

Ozier O (2018). Exploiting externalities to estimate the long-term effects of early childhood deworming. Am Econ J Appl Econ, 10(3):235–262.

Sagan A, Webb E, Azzopardi-Muscat N et al. (2021). Health systems resilience during covid-19. Lessons for building back better. United Kingdom: World Health Organization, European Commission, European Observatory on Health Systems and Policies.

Sharifi A, Pathak M, Joshi C et al. (2021). A systematic review of the health co-benefits of urban climate change adaptation. Sustain Cities Soc 74:103190.

Shaw C, Hales S, Howden-Chapman P et al. (2014). Health co-benefits of climate change mitigation policies in the transport sector. Nat Clim Chang 4(6):427–433.

Thomson S, Mosca I, Evetovits T (2020). Factsheet: Financial protection and the Sustainable Development Goals. Copenhagen (Denmark). doi: 2020-2377-42132-58027.

3 | *Politics and governance for co-benefits*

SCOTT L. GREER, MICHELLE FALKENBACH,
MATTHIAS WISMAR

3.1 Politics and governance: achieving the co-benefits

The logic of co-benefits has two compelling advantages relative to other ways of approaching intersectoral health action:

- As health policy, the causal connections between health and health systems and other outcomes are important and make a convincing case for investments in health and health policies. It also allows for an increase in attunement to the other goals health policy can influence.
- As health politics, it focuses conversations on win-win outcomes. This permits broader coalitional politics, rather than relying on the generally unproven ability of health advocates to mobilize another set of actors.

Delivering these goals, though, depends on politics governance: the institutions and organizations that make and implement decisions that can bring together or force apart organizations, sectors and people.

Achieving co-benefits puts a spotlight on politics and governance, in particular for the policy-focused approaches. How can health policymakers and health care leaders work with others to produce safe, healthy, equitable and sustainable cities and economies? How can they seek positive-sum, win-win solutions that build political coalitions to support a policy's passage, implement it, and sustain it? Such win-win approaches enhance policymakers' ability to build necessary supporting coalitions for policy (Greer et al., 2021b, 2022a).

In the previous chapter, we have identified where the impact of the co-benefits is likely. In this chapter, we address the reasons why potential win-win solutions are precluded, ignored or adopted but not implemented or sustained. Administrative history is littered with more and less successful efforts to promote "joined up government" and other such goals (Bogdanor, 2005). Here we show how we can build on these concepts to formulate and answer a set of important theoretical and practical questions.

- How can evidence from research on co-benefits be most effectively used in different political situations and systems in order to develop policies that promote co-benefits?
- What kinds of arguments and knowledge translation approaches work in different countries and political situations?
- What governance approaches work in different situations to implement and sustain co-benefits approaches?
- How should policies for co-benefits address the challenges of multi-level governance and the need for a whole of government or whole of society approach?

In health, a sector often known for its comparative isolation from the rest of government, efforts to integrate a broader logic into this argument are not new. A focus on co-benefits is an extension of longstanding research and practical experience in intersectoral policies, notably Health in All Policies (HiAP) in recent decades. The intuitions behind it are, of course, much older. Claiming that a single policy achieves multiple goals – has many co-benefits – is a persuasive tactic as old as politics. Creating or holding together a political coalition by winning supporters with different priorities is often necessary.

Governance is how societies make and implement decisions (Greer et al., 2019) – the formal and informal institutions that manage conflict and turn it into policy. This chapter introduces the two governance frameworks used throughout the case chapters to identify opportunities for action to achieve goals when political action is required.

3.2 Getting to a win-win: identifying practical co-benefits

Achieving co-benefits places the focus on *politics* and *governance*. Without them, the best-evidenced study or most persuasive model is unlikely to lead to real change. The study of political systems is rightfully a field in its own right. Everything is ultimately political, for the implications of even the most technical and scientific determinations and questions will be decided in the broad arena of politics and government (and to make something technical and scientific is to successfully constrain the scope of conflict over that topic).

This chapter presents two basic frameworks for identifying opportunities to make successful policies for co-benefits. One is for addressing the problem of change within government, in the framework commonly used by advocates of intersectoral policy. We adopt a framework from Edward C. Page that can clearly identify key dynamics and opportunities for the construction of cross-cutting policies, as well as the areas in which, under current circumstances, progress is likely to be limited and advocates might find themselves frustrated or defending their achievements against attack. This approach is essentially internal to government and the sectors involved.

The second approach to analysing politics and the possibility of action is grounded in the analysis of agenda-setting (Greer, 2015; Herweg, Zahariadis & Zöhlnhofer, 2023; Jones et al., 2016; Kingdon, 2003; Zahariadis, 2019), which has been profitably applied to the area of intersectoral policy for health (Leppo et al., 2013). Well known in health policy research, the multiple-streams framework focuses on the separate interests and development of political and policy debates as well as problems that can erupt unpredictably. The interplay of these three streams can produce a political agenda – which is not the same thing as legislation or government agreement, but is usually a precondition for any successful legislation.

In both cases, these are basic analytic frameworks for understanding which action is likely to be effective in improving the likelihood that proposals for achieving co-benefits do achieve their potential benefits. Notably, neither is a discussion of legislative adoption, a different topic that involves a wide range of institutional, partisan, economic and other factors studied by comparative politics. Nor is it a discussion of the policy design (governance of intersectoral action) and implementation after enactment. The chapter does not discuss the governance and implementation of the policies, a subject of considerable investigation and writing, which is discussed in the next chapter. Instead, the chapter focuses on two robust frameworks which can be useful in identifying opportunities to make coalitions and policies.

3.3 Salience and conflict: making policy in complex governments

Coordination is the "holy grail" of public administration (Boin et al., 2011; Peters, 2015) and the COVID-19 pandemic has clearly shown its importance (Greer et al., 2021a). Unfortunately, it is also a notoriously difficult political and administrative problem and an intractable concept for many researchers and policy thinkers. The basic problem is that the diversity of interests in any modern society means that government is pulled in many directions. While speaking of sectors or organizing around ministries and agencies gives some basic orientations to the conversation, a quick look at most health ministries shows how they often combine, or are combined with, quite diverse functions (Rose, 1987). Furthermore, organizations and institutions have entrenched interests and ways of thinking. Even if there is an argument that they could do their jobs better were they to change approaches, the process of creating widespread acceptance and implementation of a change can be very prolonged and politically exhausting.

Consider health ministries (Briatte, 2010; Greer, 2010; Mätzke, 2010; Sheard, 2010). Until the 1980s, most West European countries, Bismarck or Beveridge, folded health care into a ministry of labour or social security, packaging the delivery of health care with other areas of social insurance such as pensions and unemployment insurance. That gave health a certain kind of coherence, as a form of insurance against a social risk, but also made it hard for governments to treat health as a topic in its own right. As governments became increasingly engaged with health and health care management from the 1980s, they created freestanding health ministries along with arguments about what issues (youth? families? social care? sport?) should be packaged with and implicitly subordinated to the goals of health and health care.

Furthermore, a focus on intersectoral governance as a problem of public administration tends to direct our attention towards problems of administration when the greater challenges are often political. The recalcitrant ministry or sector will often reflect the interests of some well entrenched interest, party or faction rather than being mulish or inert. Analysts can go a long way by focusing on structural interests and politics of ministries and sectors such as transportation, health care, education or finance. However, those ministries' actions often reflect deep political disagreement rather than a problem of bureaucratic politics. Just consider the resistance of health sectors to the austerity imposed in many European countries after the 2008 financial crisis – a failure of coordination in the eyes of many finance ministries and central banks but a laudable fight to maintain essential health services in the eyes of many in the health sector (Fierlbeck, 2021; Greer & Brooks, 2020).

Hierarchy, meaning an attempt to subordinate one issue area to another, might look like a lasting solution. It is certainly a common one, with governments worldwide operating formal and informal hierarchies of departments and ministerial posts. That might be desirable, but it is unlikely to work if the underlying interests, political priorities and institutions do not support it. Instead, the solution will often lie in a more subtle politics of coalitions, identifying the particular mixtures of wins that will create a strong supportive coalition for enacting and implementing the policy. The creation of such a coalition will often depend on very specific policy compromises (for example, to do with who works or what kinds of companies provide a service) and sometimes side-deals in entirely separate areas, something generalist politicians and major interests will often do. Nonetheless, the basic social coalitions that can underpin a successful policy will often be explicable in terms of policies that unite their shared interests.

Many co-benefits can be attained by action within a single sector, ministry or organization. Improved school nutrition or reduced catastrophic health care costs can be achieved without intersectoral cooperation. They might not even require new resources if the money can be redeployed from elsewhere within the sector. This means, perhaps paradoxically, that some of the greatest co-benefits will come from sectoral, rather than intersectoral, actions. If reducing catastrophic health care costs is a route to reducing poverty and social risk, then a health care finance policy aimed at reducing it can receive support from across government. If better and more easily available school meals improve student health and education, that might be perfectly attainable within a normal education budget. Coordinating within a sector is by no means easy; it is easier to write about redeploying resources from elsewhere within the sector than to actually do it (consider the noteworthy failure of many efforts to redirect health care resources from hospitals into primary care and prevention).

It is often then harder when multiple sectors are involved, if nothing else because people within a different sector, however much they disagree, will often have a shared interest in avoiding intervention by outsiders. Understanding routes to effective action requires understanding the particular political system and government constraints involved. Fortunately, there are useful middle-range social scientific tools for this (Greer, 2022; Greer et al., 2017a, 2018). These can include understanding agenda-setting dynamics, which are useful for policy entrepreneurship and advocacy (Greer, 2015; Kingdon, 2003; Leppo et al., 2013;

	High political importance	Low political importance
High conflict	The hardest problem for intersectoral governance. Reorganization might change the parameters of conflict in a way that makes it easier to resolve, but could increase political conflict and cost.	In principle, this requires some sort of hierarchical decision. Forcing the antagonists into one common ministry might make it easier to note and resolve their conflict.
Low conflict	The second easiest kind of problem to solve. Almost any sort of intersectoral governance arrangement could, potentially, fix it.	The easiest kind of problem to solve, requiring only a hierarchical decision. Fundamentally bureaucratic problem; forcing antagonists into one common ministry might make it easier to note and resolve their divergence.

Fig. 3.1 A high salience, low conflict problem has the highest potential of being resolved

Page, 2006) as well as understanding the particular institutional and political landscape of a given country.

In terms of identifying prospects for effective action, intersectoral or within a sector, Edward C. Page developed a simple four-cell that is very useful for understanding the prospects of a proposal for action, shown in Fig. 3.1 (Page, 2005). Two questions arise when considering a proposal for action: 1) Is the proposal contentious between one or more powerful actors? 2) Is the proposal salient to high level political generalists whose intervention can force a resolution to a dispute?

In the abstract, the ideal situation for policy change is a high-salience, low-conflict policy. The second best is a low-conflict, low-salience area where patience can often achieve good outcomes. A high-conflict, low-salience issue has a bad prognosis since it is unlikely to attract the attention of more powerful actors who can decide an outcome. In contrast, a high-conflict, high-salience issue is likely to get a resolution because the top of government cannot avoid it. Note that both salience and conflict are partly rooted in the public administration and legal structures that preoccupy literature on intersectoral governance and HiAP. Still, both reflect broader politics which manifest in the creation, operation and leadership of different ministries and organizations.

The usefulness of this framework is twofold. Not only does it help to determine where a given proposal currently finds itself in terms of political importance and conflict, as previously mentioned, but it also helps us understand how the proposal can gain political importance while simultaneously becoming less conflictual. Thus, focusing on co-benefits has two potential rhetorical advantages in understanding and acting within this type of situation. First of all, it can increase the salience of the issue by offering more, or by documenting greater harms from a policy than were previously understood. For example, let's consider the impact of catastrophic health care costs as a problem of both immiseration – poverty creation – and health access. There might be a bigger constituency to address them than if we only focus on health care access. Second, focusing on co-benefits also allows us to consider ways to redirect the conversation to reduce conflict. Identifying win-win solutions can release us from win-lose (or lose-lose) policy debates that have often gone on for a very long time and are often framed entirely within the constraints of very crude budgeting logic (White, 2013). Win-win solutions are often attractive, in particular, to powerful generalist policymakers at the top, who are naturally reluctant to make tradeoffs.

3.3.1   Shaping the agenda and seizing opportunities

Almost all policy ideas seem to have been around for ever. What changes is how they are adapted to the moment by political entrepreneurs who support and advocate for them, and the mixture of policy problems and political calculations that lead to them being placed on the political agenda. This is the basic insight of the multiple-streams framework originally developed by John Kingdon, drawing on organizational studies.

The multiple streams framework is a theory of agenda-setting, not legislation (though in some systems with strong and unitary governments, the gap between being on the agenda and being adopted can be very small). It is about how a particular policy idea becomes something that is discussed and might be adopted. It focuses on three streams. The *policy* stream is where many health policy experts live. It is the discussion of policy problems and solutions. While there are many people interested in policy development and analysis, the key people involved are policy entrepreneurs who have the skills and networks, and dedicate the time, to promoting an idea and building a coalition of supporters who will validate it and aid its passage if it gets onto the agenda. Policy entrepreneurs are really a necessary condition for policies to matter. Still, they might be particularly important in the logic of co-benefits where being taken seriously across multiple policy fields requires energy and credibility in different areas that many experts will lack.

The political stream is what politicians want to do, probably summarized most simply as the need to make a mark (remember: a politician can be intensely committed to a goal, but they can best advance that goal by being in office so that politicians will prioritize election and re-election above almost anything else). The question for politicians is how a policy idea can pass and its effects – will it reward a key constituency? Will voters see, appreciate and reward it? Will it be necessary for important issues such as business confidence, unemployment or the interest rate on government debt?

Finally, the problem stream is the set of issues widely acknowledged to need a response (problems are separate from conditions, which are tacitly understood to be unchangeable and tolerated). For example, the European political agenda since 2008 has featured an economic crisis, which triggered a debt crisis; a putative refugee crisis; Brexit; a vast global pandemic with associated disruptions; and a large-scale land war. Other problems, such as geopolitical competition, economic productivity and carbon neutrality, are constantly highlighted, including regular events such as unemployment reports and fires or floods. A successful politician tries to focus their participation in this issue effectively (even if that means being unobtrusive because it isn't an issue that plays to their strengths). A successful policy entrepreneur explains how their policy contributes to solving at least one of these problems.

When the three streams come together, a policy gets on the agenda and politics can move remarkably quickly. Many of the whole of government responses to COVID-19 showed this. Co-benefits arguments might be especially well suited to getting onto the agenda since it is often easy and intellectually valid to show, for example, how health care systems can contribute to both carbon neutrality and response to disasters.

3.3.2 Credit and blame

It is almost axiomatic in political science that politicians seek to get credit for positive developments, whether or not they caused them, and avoid blame (Weaver, 1986). An abundant literature in political science discusses these dynamics (Hinterleitner, 2017, 2020) and they are key mechanisms explaining influential findings in comparative health and social policies, such as the difficulty of retrenching welfare states (Falkenbach, Bekker & Greer, 2019; Pierson, 2001). The most attractive policies are easily "traceable" for voters, designed to clarify what politician or party was responsible for the new policy or investment. In the absence of traceability, when political, fiscal or institutional constraints mean that the party or politician cannot make a traceable policy, they will often resort to "position-taking", in which they highlight their stances on major issues in lieu of being able to take creditworthy action. Traceability is also key to sustaining policies against the opposition because it clarifies which parties support and oppose a given policy. During the COVID-19 pandemic, all this behaviour was frequently on display, with heads of government centralizing government around themselves when there was credit to be had and decentralizing responsibility when blame was likely (Greer et al., 2022b), while parties unable to produce traceable, creditworthy results in health policy experimented with position-taking on issues such as masks, vaccines and China (Falkenbach & Greer, 2020).

Attention to the politics of credit and blame can lead to a distinctive approach to policymaking, advocacy and research, which differs from some common approaches. It emphasizes opportunities for clearly traceable and, therefore, simple and robustly administered policies rather than complex systems of delegation or contracting. It emphasizes policies that make the wins clear to every coalition member. It de-emphasizes arguments that complexity, such as private sector contracting, can improve efficiency or individual choice because such policies reduce traceability. It also de-emphasizes some approaches from economics. Behavioural economics arguments that focus on nudging people into good behaviour might produce the desired result but almost by definition are not traceable, and thereby less likely to produce credit or cast blame on those who would undo them. It is hard to mobilize supporters to defend a policy that was specifically designed to go unnoticed. Arguments for pricing externalities do not just create concentrated losses among, often powerful, losers, but also create more blame than credit and are therefore less attractive. Put another way, carbon pricing might be an excellent policy but subsidies for green hospitals, with the attendant jobs and grand openings, generate more credit.

3.3.3 Win-wins, coalitions and enactment

In short, the *political* appeal of co-benefits logic is that it can create new coalitions which can make new kinds of progress and policy development. It can offer different perspectives on policy from, for example,

HiAP or Healthy Cities, building on their insights as part of a more general approach that encompasses a fuller understanding of what health and health systems contribute across the board.

Coalitions are a powerful tool for analysing politics and policies, and a strong coalition that can support a policy can be strengthened by that policy and help support its implementation. Developing governance to do that is crucial, and the subject of the next chapter.

3.4   Governance: overcoming challenges of implementation and sustainability

Implementation is famously one of the most theoretically and empirically challenging topics in social sciences. It is not for want of attention by researchers in fields as diverse as public administration, political science, economics, change management, organizational behaviour and psychology. There are powerful reasons why something that has been decided might be ignored at the level where it must be implemented – from habit to complexity to inadequate resources to poor communications to interest group resistance to corruption to well founded disagreement with the policy. It appears that, for all the effort, there is no one good theory of implementation or how it works which can be adopted across different contexts (a sign of this is the burgeoning new field of implementation science).

A second question is how to sustain, or entrench, a policy over time. Sustainability is a second question of great interest to political science researchers but often receives less attention in public health and health policy literatures (Greer & Lillvis, 2014). Put simply, most officials, ministers and governments are not in position long enough to assume that even the policies they implement will be sustained. New officials, ministers and governments will have their own agendas, might be actively hostile to their predecessor's activities, and are often unlikely to invest too much energy in the previous agenda. Interest groups and others who lost out on the original decision and resisted implementation will have additional opportunities to undermine the policy. We can see this in some of the most dramatic policies the EU has adopted in the twenty-first century as well as endless examples in government.

There is a variety of solutions that governments can adopt in trying to address the sustainability problem and entrench their programmes. They include entrenching them in legislation or even constitutional law, the effectiveness of which varies with political institutions. The more difficult it is to legislate, the more value politicians will see in legislation since the difficulty of legislating will deter or defeat successors who do not value the policy. They also can include mandatory requirements of various sorts, which expand the scope of conflict and thereby make it harder for governments to renege on commitments. This can mean, for example, mandatory submission of reports on progress to the legislature, publication of regular and relevant data, and public consultation processes which allow allies in civil society to follow policy closely and argue for continued policy implementation. They include public visibility and "traceability" of benefits, allowing voters to know who, and what policy, is responsible for something good they received. They can also include the legal system's use, for example, in the form of rights of action that can be enforced through lawsuits. This is partly achieved through simple policy design, which makes it clear where benefits and co-benefits come from.

Progress and sustainability require governance, which is the set of processes by which decisions are made and implemented (Greer et al., 2016, 2019). To some extent governance in a country is usually a given; there are legal, bureaucratic, political, cultural and other limits to how much any particular policy area or programme is likely to diverge from how things are generally done in a country. But governance is constantly changing, being reshaped by political and institutional evolution as well as the policies themselves, whose organization changes "the way things are done" for the future.

The TAPIC framework (Box 3.1) is a useful analytical tool for identifying problems in governance (Greer, Wismar & Figueras, 2015). The framework first determines whether a problem can be attributed to governance (as against, for example, inadequate resources) and then identifies the particular governance problem: transparency, accountability, participation, integrity and policy capacity.

If we assume that the case for a particular programme with co-benefits has been made, then the question is what mechanisms will promote the necessary level of intersectoral governance. Longer discussions can be found in Greer, Wismar and Figueras (2016), and especially Lillvis and Greer (2016) and McQueen and colleagues (2012). Table 3.1 is a schematic presentation of the below described approaches, drawing on and expanding the more structural (organizational and budgetary) approach developed in earlier work (McQueen et al., 2012).

Box 3.1 TAPIC: the five domains of governance

Transparency means that institutions inform the public and other actors of both upcoming decisions and decisions that have been made, and of the process by and grounds on which decisions are being made.

Accountability means that an actor must give an account of its actions, with consequences if the action and explanation are inadequate.

Participation means that affected parties have an opportunity to provide input to relevant deliberations without fear of retribution.

Integrity means that the processes of representation, decisionmaking, employment and enforcement should be clearly specified. Individuals and organizations should have a clear allocation of roles and responsibilities.

Policy capacity refers to the ability to develop policy that is aligned with resources in pursuit of goals.

Sources: Greer, Vasev & Wismar, 2017; Greer et al., 2019

Table 3.1 *Framework for governance tools and actions*

Category	Tool	Possible governance actions with these tools
Plan		
	Plan	Goals and targets, policy guidance, financial support, legal mandate
Indicators and targets		
	Indicator	Evidence support, monitoring and evaluation
	Target	Goals and targets, monitoring and evaluation
Budgeting		
	Pooled budget	Goals and targets, financial support, implementation and management
	Shared objectives	Goals and targets, financial support, implementation and management

Table 3.1 *(Cont.)*

Category	Tool	Possible governance actions with these tools
Organization	Coordinated budgeting	Goals and targets, financial support, implementation and management
	Ministerial linkages	Coordination, policy guidance, financial support, implementation and management
	Specific ministers	Coordination, monitoring and evaluation, policy guidance, implementation and management
	Legislative committees	Evidence support, advocacy, monitoring and evaluation, implementation and management
	Interdepartmental committees/units	Evidence support, coordination, monitoring and evaluation, policy guidance, implementation and management
	Departmental mergers	Coordination, policy guidance, financial support, implementation and management
Accountability	Engagement (e.g., civil society, industry, public)	Evidence support, advocacy, monitoring and evaluation, implementation and management
	Transparent data	Evidence support, advocacy, monitoring and evaluation
	Regular reporting	Evidence support, advocacy, monitoring and evaluation
	Independent agency/ evaluators	Evidence support, advocacy, monitoring and evaluation
	Support for civil society	Evidence support, advocacy, monitoring and evaluation
	Legal rights	Advocacy, monitoring and evaluation, legal mandate

3.4.1 Plans

One of the conceptually simplest ways to implement co-benefits is to start with a plan. A plan chooses some coherent goals and identifies the resources and actions needed to achieve them – for example, the changes to health financing and access and surrounding social provision that would be required to reduce the contribution of ill health to poverty, or the changes to the actions of health sector employers needed to remove discrimination. A plan can be a necessary requirement for action, and the planning process can also be a valuable way of connecting organizations and identifying resources and possibilities. Still, it will only work if it has consistent political support, some attention to the interests of the involved actors and, ideally, both high salience and low conflict.

3.4.2 *Indicators and Targets*

Gathering data is an important part of identifying, let alone addressing, a problem. A large part of the SDGs programme involves finding and improving indicators that let countries, their citizens and the world view their progress and challenges. The SDG indicators enterprise can be critiqued, as is to be expected of something so complex and global, but it is nonetheless ambitious and important. Indicators are measures of particular broader phenomena, such as infant mortality or employment discrimination, and are often constructed in subtle ways from other, more basic data (for example, infant mortality statistics rest on a foundation of birth and death statistics that required decades of political argument to establish in even rich countries). We can use indicators to identify broad issues, ideally unobtrusive ones that are less likely to be gamed. An indicator is not a target: as soon as an indicator becomes a target, it ceases to be an indicator (Campbell, 1979; Goodhart, 1984). That is because the more important a measure, the more likely it is to be manipulated – the dark side of the saying that "what's measured is what's managed". Thus, the SDGs are goals but the indicators are less likely to be gamed because of their sheer profusion.

One way to proceed might be to focus on developing and using a mixture of robust and, if possible, unobtrusive measures (Webb et al., 1999) from multiple areas to understand progress towards overarching goals such as the SDGs. Another is to use the SDGs as leverage to broaden goals, targets and indicators taken into account in policy.

3.4.3   Budgets

Budgets set and reflect organizations' priorities, and budgeting tools are therefore a key instrument used by policymakers to direct activity towards co-benefits. There is a well established public financial management literature and approach which starts with a conceptual description of the budgeting process framed in stages, namely planning (determining the relationship between goals and expenditures), budgeting (mapping available resources onto specific budget lines) and monitoring (ensuring that budgeted funds are spent in the most appropriate way). Each stage has more subdivisions, but they broadly map how governments and other organizations budget and identify opportunities to improve practice.

In this context, budgeting techniques for intersectoral action include: pooled budget; shared accountability, goals and outcomes; or coordinated budgeting (often informally, in the manner of ministerial linkages, discussed below). It is important to underscore that in budgeting, as well as any other activity, evaluation and monitoring are crucial and need to be built into the policy design from the start. Otherwise, it will be difficult to tell what, if anything, was achieved.

3.4.4   Organizations

Reorganization and organization are another key tool used to achieve intersectoral action and effects. There are many ways to reshape government organizations, and many limitations on the effects (Greer, 2010; Mätzke, 2011). These can include (Greer, Wismar & Figueras, 2016; McQueen et al., 2012): ministerial linkages (such as small teams of cabinet ministers), specific ministers (for example, for public health or equity), special parliamentary committees to raise awareness and keep government accountable, interdepartmental committees and units, mergers (for example, of health and sport or justice and equity), or specific efforts to engage the public and stakeholders such as industry. In each of these cases, it is crucial to understand the context and formulate a goal relevant to the salience, importance and goals of the different actors. When there is agreement on a goal, but no agreement on the best methods of achieving it, and a highly unattractive alternative to achieving the goal, for example, it is relatively easy for organizations to work together (low conflict-high salience) (Sabel & Zeitlin, 2007, 2010), but in other cases a more hierarchical approach might be more useful.

3.4.5 People

Policy analysts and public administration students, focused on developing policies that will be resilient to future incompetent or weak staff, often downplay the importance of people. Politicians and policymakers, by contrast, often adhere to the idea that "personnel is policy" – that appointing the right people can be a far more effective strategy than changing structures or budgeting rules. That is because people can lead – set agendas and priorities within and around their organization – while also using their discretion to advance the agenda through decisions about programmes, research, staffing, pilots, evaluations and budgetary proposals. Networks of people with shared convictions can be extremely effective, as a great deal of research has shown, and advocates of co-benefits can ensure that interested politicians will have access to capable staff who understand the issues.

The implication is that time-honoured techniques of developing skills, awareness and training in managers, policymakers, analysts and staff should not be neglected, and investment in training them in the policy analysis and evaluation techniques for intersectoral governance can be richly rewarded. Furthermore, encouraging cross-sectoral professional networks (which go by many names in the social sciences (Greer & Löblová, 2020; Löblová, 2018) means that it is possible for an engaged politician or senior policymaker to find a group of potential allies who can inform policy and carry out the work. A minister with no policy capacity – which means capable people – will quickly find the limits of political will (Greer et al., 2016).

3.4.6 Accountability

One of the key problems of implementation and, especially, sustainability, is accountability. Ministers leave, prime ministers leave and governments leave. Agendas change – over the last decade, European political agendas have bounced from one crisis to another (climate change, economic crisis, refugee "crisis", COVID-19 and now the Russian invasion of Ukraine). How do strategic policymakers ensure that there will be accountability for delivering outcomes after they have gone?

One technique is to act, while in office, to strengthen outside accountability for those goals (Greer & Lillvis, 2014). Thus, for example, legislating mandatory reports to the legislature and public on progress;

creating oversight and watchdog agencies and evaluators that can report on failure; mandating the collection and public release of relevant data; joining international collaborations that require benchmarking and data reporting; and even requiring particular public reports are all ways to enhance accountability by making it easier for civil society, the media, researchers, politicians and legislators to know when a government is faltering and put pressure on it (Greer et al., 2017b). Even if subsequent governments try to reverse these mechanisms by defunding activists or interfering with data collection, as they often will (Rocco et al., 2021), that creates new opportunities to call them to account. Finally, the courts can be used to create accountability by creating a right of action – the ability for somebody to file suit against the government or other public agencies if they fail to take broader co-benefits into account. This is a tool governments are often hesitant to deploy, but it can be powerful.

3.4.7   Summary

Table 3.1 shows the different options in what is inevitably an incomplete list of options. It shows some of the commonly used tools of intersectoral action and the purposes to which they are put.

The chapters in this book use this framework to categorize different mechanisms. While the list is necessarily always incomplete, it can contribute to understanding what worked and what kinds of options exist if we are to institutionalize intersectoral governance that attains co-benefits.

3.5   Conclusion

Governance and politics in the abstract are not always interesting or productive topics, but figuring out the political coalitions' governance arrangements that will create and sustain intersectoral co-benefits is complex and vitally important. How do the law and organization of each sector contribute to or impede intersectoral action? What policy tools might help to change that?

In particular, intersectoral action faces the twin challenges of implementation and sustainability. Implementation challenges receive much of the attention in policy debates and literature, since it is clear that many statements of intersectoral good intentions, like many policies of all kind, do not turn into real changes. There are many ways policymakers approach the implementation problem, as shown in Table 3.1, which can include budget, procedural and other changes to the way policy is made, substantive plans and targets, and appointments of key people.

But politicians and policymakers also must focus on the sustainability of their approaches. Enactment of a policy creates new challenges and might give opponents new opportunities to delay or reverse changes, while also creating the possibility of policy that can win supporters as it is implemented. Policymakers meet the sustainability challenge by identifying ways to entrench intersectorality through techniques as different as reporting to the legislature, creating legal rights, and developing internal review processes within government. Entrenching policy is urgent because otherwise bureaucratic entropy combines with political opposition to undermine that policy. It is also a kind of political thinking, because it involves anticipating potential supporters who can defend and extend the policy once the ministers are long out of office, and identifying ways to empower them.

Governance for co-benefits, in particular, is often going to be about supporting coalitions of different interests which can support each other even after a government decides it is time to go back to basics (for example, not focusing on win-win solutions and instead focusing on a few targets), changes ideological orientation, or simply loses interest. Fortunately, the vocabulary and range of international experience means that there is a great deal of writing and thought in this area, and it shows the importance of creating and entrenching coalitions. That, of course, is best done with a win-win approach.

References

Bogdanor V (ed.). (2005). Joined-up Government. Oxford: British Academy/ Oxford University Press.

Boin A, Ansell C, Lodge M et al. (2011). A time for public administration. Public Adm, 89(2):221–225.

Briatte F (2010). A Case of Weak Architecture: The French Ministry of Health. Soc Policy Adm, 44(2):155–170.

Campbell DT (1979). Assessing the impact of planned social change. Evaluation and program planning, 2(1):67–90.

Falkenbach M, Greer SL (2020). Denial and Distraction: How the Populist Radical Right Responds to COVID-19 Comment on "A Scoping Review of PRR Parties' Influence on Welfare Policy and its Implication for Population Health in Europe". Int J Health Policy Manag., 10(9):578–580.

Falkenbach M, Bekker M, Greer SL (2019). Do parties make a difference? A review of partisan effects on health and the welfare state. Eur J Public Health, 30(4):673–682.

Fierlbeck K (2021). Health Care and the Fate of Social Europe. J Health Polit Policy Law, 46(1):1–22. doi:10.1215/03616878-8706579.

Goodhart CAE (1984). Problems of monetary management: the UK experience. In: Goodhart CAE (ed.) Monetary Theory and Practice. London: Red Globe Press; 91–121.

Greer SL (2010). Editorial Introduction: Health Departments in Health Policy. Soc Policy Adm, 44(2):113–119.

Greer SL (2015). John W. Kingdon, Agendas, Alternatives, and Public Policy. In: Balla SJ, Lodge M, Page EC (eds) The Oxford Handbook of Classics in Public Policy and Administration. Oxford University Press; 417–432.

Greer SL (2022). Professions, Data, and Political Will: From the Pandemic Toward a Political Science with Public Health. In: Fafard P, de Leeuw E, Cassola A (eds) Integrating Science and Politics for Public Health (33–57). Springer Open Access. (https://link.springer.com/chapter/10.1007/978-3-030-98985-9_3)

Greer SL, Brooks E (2020). Termites of Solidarity in the House of Austerity: Undermining Fiscal Governance in the European Union. [8706615]. J Health Polit Policy Law, 46(1):71–92. doi:10.1215/03616878-8706615.

Greer SL, Lillvis DF (2014). Beyond leadership: political strategies for coordination in health policies. Health Policy, 116(1):12–17. doi:10.1016/j.healthpol.2014.01.019.

Greer SL, Löblová O (2020). Networks after Brexit. In: Laible J, Greer SL (eds) The European Union after Brexit. Manchester University Press; 146–161.

Greer SL, Vasev N, Wismar M (2017). Fences and ambulances: Intersectoral governance for health. Health Policy, 121(11):1101–1104.

Greer SL, Wismar M, Figueras J (2015). EBOOK: Strengthening health system governance: better policies, stronger performance. McGraw-Hill Education (UK).

Greer SL, Wismar M, Figueras J (2016). Strengthening health system governance: better policies, stronger performance. Brussels/Philadelphia: European Observatory on Health Systems and Policies/Open University Press.

Greer SL, Wismar M, Figueras J et al. (2016). Governance: a framework. In: Greer SL, Wismar M, Figueras J (eds) Strengthening Health System Governance. Open University Press; 27–56.

Greer SL, Bekker M, de Leeuw E et al. (2017a). Policy, politics and public health. Eur J Public Health, 27(4):40–43.

Greer SL, Wismar M, Pastorino G et al. (eds). (2017b). Civil Society and Health: Contributions and Potential. Brussels: European Observatory on Health Systems and Policies.

Greer SL, Bekker MPM, Azzopardi-Muscat N et al. (2018). Political analysis in public health: middle-range concepts to make sense of the politics of health. Eur J Public Health, 28(suppl_3):3–6. doi:10.1093/eurpub/cky159.

Greer SL, Vasev N, Jarman H et al. (2019). It's the governance, stupid! TAPIC: A governance framework to strengthen decision making and implementation. Copenhagen: European Observatory on Health Systems and Policies.

Greer SL, Jarman H, Falkenbach M et al. (2021a). Social policy as an integral component of pandemic response: Learning from COVID-19 in Brazil, Germany, India and the United States. Glob Public Health, 16(8–9):1209–1222.

Greer SL, Lynch JF, Reeves A et al. (2021b). The Politics of Healthy Ageing. Cambridge: Cambridge University Press.

Greer SL, Lynch JF, Reeves A et al. (2022a). The politics of healthy ageing: myths and realities. Brussels: European Observatory on Health Systems and Policies.

Greer SL, Rozenblum S, Falkenbach M et al. (2022b). Centralizing and decentralizing governance in the COVID-19 pandemic: The politics of credit and blame. Health Policy, 126(5):408–417.

Herweg N, Zahariadis N, Zohlnhöfer R (2023). The Multiple Streams Framework: Foundations, Refinements, and Empirical Applications." In Weible CM (ed.) Theories of the Policy Process, 5th edn (New York: Routledge), 29–64.

Hinterleitner M (2017). Reconciling Perspectives on Blame Avoidance Behaviour. Political Stud Rev, 15(2):243–254. doi:10.1111/1478-9302.12099.

Hinterleitner M (2020). Policy Controversies and Political Blame Games. Cambridge: Cambridge University Press. doi:10.1017/9781108860116.

Jones MD, Peterson HL, Pierce JJ et al. (2016). A River Runs Through It: A Multiple Streams Meta-Review. Policy Stud J, 44(1):13–36. doi:10.1111/psj.12115.

Kingdon JW (2003). Agendas, Alternatives, and Public Policies. New York: HarperCollins.

Leppo K, Ollila E, Peña S et al. (eds). (2013). Health in All Policies – Seizing opportunities, implementing policies. European Observatory on Health Systems and Policies/Sosiaali-ja terveysministerio (STM).

Lillvis DF, Greer SL (2016). Strategies for policy success: Achieving 'good' governance. In: Greer SL, Wismar M, Figueras J (eds) Strengthening Health System Governance: Better Policies, Stronger Performance. Maidenhead: Open University Press; 57–84.

Löblová O (2018). Epistemic communities and experts in health policy-making. Eur J Public Health, 28(suppl_3):7–10. doi:10.1093/eurpub/cky156.

McQueen D, Wismar M, Lin V et al. (2012). Introduction: Health in All Policies, the social determinants of health and governance. In: McQueen D, Wismar M, Lin V et al. (eds) Inter-sectoral Governance for Health in All Policies: Structures, actions and experiences. Copenhagen: WHO Regional Office for Europe/European Observatory on Health Systems and Policies.

McQueen D, Wismar M, Lin V et al. (eds) (2012). Inter-sectoral Governance for Health in All Policies: Structures, actions and experiences. Copenhagen: WHO Regional Office for Europe/European Observatory on Health Systems and Policies.

Mätzke M (2010). The organization of health policy functions in the German Federal Government. Soc Policy Adm, 44(2):120–141.

Mätzke M (2011). Political Competition and Unequal Social Rights. J Public Policy, 31(1):1–24. doi:10.1017/S0143814X1000022X.

Page EC (2005). Joined-Up Government and the Civil Service. In: Bogdanor V (ed.) Joined-Up Government. Oxford: Oxford University Press/British Academy; 139–155.

Page EC (2006). The Origins of Policy. In: Moran M, Rein M, Goodin RE (eds) The Oxford Handbook of Public Policy. Oxford: Oxford University Press; 207–226.

Peters BG (2015). Policy capacity in public administration. Policy Soc, 34(3–4):219–228.

Pierson P (2001). The New Politics of the Welfare State. Oxford: Oxford University Press.

Rocco P, Rich JA, Klasa J et al. (2021). Who Counts Where? COVID-19 Surveillance in Federal Countries. J Health Polit Policy Law, 46(6):959–987.

Rose R (1987). Ministers and Ministries: A Functional Analysis. Oxford: Clarendon.

Sabel CF, Zeitlin J (2007). Learning from Difference: The New Architecture of Experimentalist Governance in the European Union. Eur Law J, 14(3):271–327.

Sabel CF, Zeitlin J (eds). (2010). Experimentalist Governance in the European Union: Towards a New Architecture. Oxford: Oxford University Press.

Sheard S (2010). Quacks and Clerks: Historical and Contemporary Perspectives on the Structure and Function of the British Medical Civil Service. Soc Policy Adm, 44(2):193–207.

Ståhl T, Wismar M, Ollila E et al. (eds). (2006). Health in all policies: prospects and potentials. Finland: Ministry of Social Affairs and Health.

Weaver RK (1986). The Politics of Blame Avoidance. J Public Policy, 6:371–398.

Webb EJ, Campbell DT, Schwartz RD et al. (1999). Unobtrusive Measures. SAGE Publications. (https://books.google.com/books?id=vhF1AwAAQBAJ)

White J (2013). Budget-makers and health care systems. Health Policy, 112(3):163–171.

Zahariadis N (2019). The multiple streams framework: Structure, limitations, prospects. In: Sabatier P (ed.,) Theories of the Policy Process (New York: Routledge), 65–92.

4 | *Next steps: making Health for All Policies*

SCOTT L. GREER, MICHELLE FALKENBACH,
MATTHIAS WISMAR

4.1 Introduction

The case for Health for All Policies is not just that other policies can affect health – it is that health can contribute to the achievement of a wide range of policy goals, from avoiding catastrophic costs that push people into poverty, to reducing gender inequalities in work, to reducing climate change and enhancing urban environments.

This is a summons to generalist policymakers and governments not to underestimate the impact of health expenditures on their economies and societies. Better health can lead to better education, work and equality, among many other things, while health expenditure, intelligently used, can lead to scientific and industrial development, workforce investment, and more liveable and sustainable cities. Investment in health and better health outcomes clearly contribute to economic growth. Understanding the impact of better health across the SDGs can show the importance of a focus on better health outcomes.

This is also a summons to health sector policymakers. The policy and scholarly literature on Health in All Policies is vast. We found in our research that there was far less attention paid to what health policies and organizations could do for others – to the ways in which health policies, focused on health outcomes, can contribute to avoidable problems ranging from global heating to unsustainable cities to inequalities in the workforce. Health *for* All Policies does not just rebrand Health in All Policies with a new look; it also calls on policymakers, and people across the health sector, to do what they have called on others to do and think about the impact of their decisions on the rest of society – which as we all know, will eventually also affect health.

4.2 Understanding co-benefits

This book's substantive chapters present variations on a methodological approach that could be used and improved in scholarly and policy research. The book identified, in Chapter 1, two causal mechanisms connecting health policies and systems with achieving other goals. One is through the actions of health policies and systems directly; the other is through improved health status. The two approaches require different kinds of policy analysis to develop. Still, in both cases there is ample scope to create precise and persuasive policy analysis that can identify areas where health policy and health can help to achieve other goals.

In the substantive chapters of this book, we focus on how *health policies and systems* can contribute to the other SDGs, in their capacities as employers, research-intensive industries, large owners of infrastructure, expensive services, businesses, and more. This is an often under-appreciated area of study. For all that health policy analysts and advocates, under the flag of HiAP, called for health to be a focus of other policy areas, health policies and systems did not always contribute what they could. The low-hanging fruit that is so easy to see in other sectors, the walkable streets unbuilt or the healthy school food unserved, was replicated in the city-centre hospitals unbuilt or the industrial food purchases of the hospital. In other words, part of Health for All Policies means developing the policy analysis tools to understand the impact of health infrastructure and services on climate change and cities, or the impact of the health care sector's employment decisions on jobs and inequalities. The COVID-19 pandemic briefly made public health policy exceptionally important. It also showed the importance of integrating broader public policy with health in a way that went far beyond pre-crisis concepts of intersectoral action (Greer et al., 2021a; Jarman, 2021).

Researching this topic would follow the model of the substantive chapters. Starting with knowledge of the specific topic area, it would involve identifying the key mechanisms through which health policies and systems affect other SDGs and the policy tools available which could change that impact for the better. It would then be subject to filtering what is possible, not just in the abstract but in the concrete political situation and governance arrangements. As a side benefit, if this identified problems (for example in government contracting rules or accountability arrangements) which prevented health policies and systems from contributing to broader win-win outcomes, that would be an insight of use for reforming governance in a way that otherwise might not emerge.

A second approach, equally important, would be to develop and improve methods for estimating the impact on other SDGs of *improved health status*. This would build on existing literature, discussed in Chapters 1 and 2, that finds a positive relationship between improved health and education, employment, economic growth and other SDG goals. The possibilities for finding and using data are endless, and the consequences of developing and diffusing tools and estimates of the impact of improved health on other policy areas could be dramatic.

In both, it is important to emphasize the importance of reducing health inequalities. Many SDGs contain specific discussions of the importance of equity, and some are specifically about it. The need to address inequalities in order to address overall social goods is a basic mathematical as well as an ethical proposition. One way to shift an average result is to try to shift the median person in the distribution; another is to look and see if something is producing fat tails of people who are suffering needlessly. If a health inequality, such as failing to address any single population's needs, is shaping overall health outcomes, then it might be an efficient way to improve health for the whole population as well as an imperative to redress inequalities.

It is also important to underline the role of politics and governance analysis in both the development of policies and the development of tools for policy analysis. The challenges of intersectoral governance in the case of HiAP are well known. Still, there is scope to reframe the question as: what political conditions and governance arrangements enable H4AP, through the identification and enactment of win-win, positive-sum policies? In terms of broader governance, are there specific policies in areas such as legislative organization, budgeting processes and rules, or legal accountability, which impede win-win solutions and how might they be changed?

4.3   Attaining co-benefits: politics

Co-benefits are, in principle, a way to turn zero-sum conversations about budgets and political priority into a focus on win-win solutions. The allocation of money, authority, credit and blame will have to be negotiated over and over again between policymakers and other groups. Still, the potential benefits across government can be dramatic. Nonetheless, there will be resistance in different contexts.

One of the ways in which political processes can be redirected to identify co-benefits is to mainstream such thinking in the various units of government engaged in policy analysis and evaluation. These units, typically found across government and most powerful in units associated with finance ministries and heads of government, can often shape government action with superficially technical discussions of cost-benefit, cost-effectiveness and other kinds of evaluations. While understanding the mixture of economics, accounting and modelling that these practitioners do can be a challenge, it is often crucial to those who would advocate for a policy change built on the subtler and more interconnected logic of co-benefits. One approach is to extend the diversity and complexity of their models, by, for example, paying more attention to the externalities of a policy (consider, once again, the impact on other SDGs of a new-build hospital on the edge of the city with poor public transport). Basic methods such as attributing quality-adjusted life years (QALYs) can, in principle, be applied to the impact of policies far beyond health technology. Another is to consider additional endpoints, such as wellness, happiness, human development or even a conceptually simple focus on lives saved by different interventions.

The European Union, in particular, has declared that the SDGs are the goals of its Semester, replacing its older 2020 goals (Greer & Brooks, 2020; Greer et al., 2022; Verdun & Vanhercke, 2022). This decision by the EU is not just an impressive change from the Semester's early and intense focus on deficits. It also creates a potential opportunity to use the Semester, a large and increasingly sophisticated process, to expand the range of commonly used analytic techniques that governments use in order to show how policies attain more than one SDG through co-benefits.

The politics of knowledge are important, and we might be surprised how many policies look different and can be evaluated differently if we have better accepted ways of analysing co-benefits. But there are also straightforward politics. Most existing activities of government come with constituencies that have strong interests in something like a better-funded version of the status quo. From professions to pharmaceutical companies, health is no exception at all to this rule. But the political hope of a logic of co-benefits is that it can create different coalitions – by, for example, changing the scope of conflict surrounding decisions about health infrastructure, employment, research and other topics (Hacker & Pierson, 2014; Schattschneider, 1935).

4.4   Implementing and sustaining co-benefits: governance

While every situation and place is different, there are consistent problems in implementing and sustaining policy change, problems which are made worse in intersectoral contexts where concepts, priorities, interests and all manner of organizational, legal and infrastructural legacies shape what can be done. Part of the logic of co-benefits is that it can create or reform coalitions, by, for example, showing how the size and type of resources invested in the health sector can attain other goals through better health or through health policies and systems. Nonetheless, it is important to focus on the governance that can lead organizations to actually implement new priorities and keep implementing them even after the politics have changed. How do we construct, in short, governance that supports Health for All Policies?

Table 3.1 lists a number of the key ways policymakers have tried to support intersectoral governance, including budgets, appointments, plans and laws. Each has its place, but it is often important to focus on ways to entrench policies through legislation and budgetary processes, as well as review and evaluation systems, which make clear their value and are hard to change.

4.5   Conclusion: key takeaways

The Health in All Policies (HiAP) approach was often alive to the political and practical advantages of positive-sum, win-win policies but often was read as emphasizing a one-directional relationship between health and other sectors (transport, environment, education and health) to produce positive health outcomes. Examples of this include better street designs to promote the use of bicycles, and more nutritious foods in schools leading to fewer health problems. The result was two significant problems with the HiAP approach. The first is that it has proven difficult to engage other sectors as they are likely convinced that health ministers expect other sectors to fix their problems. The second problem is that many sectors believe health is not their business (de Leeuw, 2017).

While the second problem was partially solved during the COVID-19 pandemic in which sectors were forced to work together in the name of health, the issue of sustainability remains. How can we get sectors to work together over time (Greer & Lillvis, 2014)? We argue that creating co-benefits for multiple sectors across shared goals can be the answer. Thus, rather than reinvent the idea of HiAP, we propose that it simply needs to be expanded. Instead of just offering the one-directional relationship that HiAP proposes (other sectors ➔ health), an expansion of thought is required to make this offer two-dimensional. Health for All Policies posits that other sectors help the health sector, and that the health sector helps other sectors. This new relationship highlights what health can do for other sectors while simultaneously attaining co-benefits for its own sector.

The takeaways from this project can be summarized this way:

- Move from Health in All Policies to Health *for* All Policies. This proposes keeping the already existing relationship between health and other sectors and the health co-benefits they produce and adding a new relationship that puts other sectors at the forefront and highlights what they can do for health whilst simultaneously attaining co-benefits for their sectors.
- There are three reasons to focus on co-benefits if we are to achieve the SDG target goals: co-benefits for other sectors of health policy and investment can open up new policy opportunities; co-benefits are likely to be necessary if we are to attain key goals; and interacting sources of health and health inequalities can be better understood.
- Achieving co-benefits places the focus on politics. Without the cooperation of political actors, proposals remain ideas instead of becoming concrete actions or policies. Often, when the focus is placed on politics we are faced with a political problem, namely that the government does not agree with itself.
- Intersectoral governance structures are important to consider when attempting to address and achieve the targets laid out within the SDGs. By aligning both health and non-health objectives, co-benefits can be achieved. This benefits not only the health sector, but also any other sector (environment, education, transportation, etc.) working in unison with the health sector.

The time is right to reconsider intersectoral – and sectoral – action for broad goals. COVID-19 showed that governments worldwide, poor and rich, are capable of extraordinary policy and integration feats (Greer et al., 2021a). It showed the interconnections of many policy sectors and ruthlessly exposed weaknesses of all kinds (Sagan et al., 2021). It created interest in future work to build the resilience of health systems and societies (Hynes et al., 2020; McKee, 2021; Williamson et al., 2022). And, in terms of the SDGs, it also did tremendous damage. The impact of the pandemic on health, directly and indirectly, was a disaster for much of the world (WHO, 2022). The interaction of the pandemic and various social, economic and policy responses reversed the already faltering progress the world was making on many other SDGs (United Nations, Sustainable Development Goals Report 2021). A pre-pandemic debate about whether we were making sufficient progress has turned into a post-pandemic debate about whether we can ever make up the regress and start to make gains again. Without Health for All Policies, the answer might well be no.

References

De Leeuw E (2017). Engagement of sectors other than health in integrated health governance, policy, and action. Annu Rev Public Health, 38:329–349.

Greer SL, Brooks E (2020). Termites of Solidarity in the House of Austerity: Undermining Fiscal Governance in the European Union. [8706615]. J Health Polit Policy Law, 46(1):71–92. doi:10.1215/03616878-8706615.

Greer SL, Lillvis DF (2014). Beyond leadership: political strategies for coordination in health policies. Health Policy, 116(1):12–17. doi:10.1016/j.healthpol.2014.01.019.

Greer SL, Jarman H, Falkenbach M et al. (2021a). Social policy as an integral component of pandemic response: Learning from COVID-19 in Brazil, Germany, India and the United States. Glob Public Health, 16(8–9):1209–1222.

Greer SL, King EJ, da Fonseca EM et al. (eds). (2021b). Coronavirus Politics: The Comparative Politics and Policy of COVID-19. Ann Arbor: University of Michigan Press.

Greer SL, Rozenblum S, Fahy N et al. (2022). Everything you always wanted to know about European Union health policy but were afraid to ask (3rd, completely revised ed.). Brussels: WHO/European Observatory on Health Systems and Policies.

Hacker JS, Pierson P (2014). After the "master theory": Downs, Schattschneider, and the rebirth of policy-focused analysis. Perspect Politics, 12(3):643–662.

Hynes W, Trump B, Love P et al. (2020). Bouncing forward: a resilience approach to dealing with COVID-19 and future systemic shocks. Environ Syst Decis, 40(2):174–184.

Jarman H (2021). State Responses to the COVID-19 Pandemic: Governance, Surveillance, Coercion and Social Policy. In Greer SL, King EJ, da Fonseca EM et al. (eds). Coronavirus Politics: The Comparative Politics and Policy of COVID-19. Ann Arbor: University of Michigan Press.

McKee M (ed.). (2021). Drawing light from the pandemic: a new strategy for health and sustainable development. A review of the evidence. Brussels: European Observatory on Health Systems and Policies.

Sagan A, Webb E, Azzopardi-Muscat N et al. (2021). Health systems resilience during covid-19. Lessons for building back better. United Kingdom: World Health Organization, European Commission, European Observatory on Health Systems and Policies.

Schattschneider EE (1935). Politics, Pressures, and the Tariff. New York: Prentice Hall.

United Nations. Sustainable Development Goals Report 2021. United Nations.

Verdun A, Vanhercke B (2022). Are (some) social players entering European recovery through the Semester back door. In: Vanhercke B, Spasova S (eds) Social policy in the European Union: state of play 2021. ETUI, The European Trade Union Institute; 107–130.

Williamson A, Forman R, Azzopardi-Muscat N et al. (2022). Effective post-pandemic governance must focus on shared challenges. Lancet, 399(10340):199–2001.

WHO (2022). World health statistics 2022: monitoring health for the SDGs, sustainable development goals.

5 | SDG1, eliminating poverty: improvements to health coverage design as a means to create co-benefits between health system and poverty Sustainable Development Goals

BILLY DERING, MICHELLE FALKENBACH, JON CYLUS

5.1 Introduction

Poverty is often defined as an inability to meet basic needs for human survival and certain normal activities (Ravallion, 2010). Poverty reduction is a top priority of governments around the world, with 'Ending poverty in all its forms everywhere' as Goal 1 of the UN Sustainable Development Goals (SDGs).

To address poverty, one must be able to measure it. This is typically done by assessing how many people are living below a poverty line representing some basic standard of living. While the international poverty line is often defined as living on $1.90 per person per day, there is no universal poverty line in use and a range of poverty lines are used in practice depending on the national setting (United Nations, 2022). A distinction is made between absolute poverty lines, defined by a fixed monetary amount, and relative poverty lines that can vary depending on the average income level of the economy in which one resides. The absolute poverty definition is most commonly used in low- and middle-income countries, while relative poverty is mostly used in high-income settings. Regardless of the poverty line used, the aim of measuring poverty is the same: identifying those who experience severe financial hardship.

To make progress on SDG Goal 1, policymakers must address a wide range of causes of poverty, including economic, social and political factors. Health and health systems also play an important role. For example, people in poor health may be unable to work, and, as we have seen in recent years, communicable diseases such as COVID-19 can lead to economic disruption.

Health systems can also influence the risk of poverty through exposure to out-of-pocket payments, which are payments for health care goods and services made at the point of use. According to global estimates from the World Bank, almost 90 million people each year fall into poverty due to out-of-pocket spending on health care (World Bank, 2021). Many others experience high levels of out-of-pocket health spending relative to their available financial resources – so-called catastrophic payments – that, while not necessarily causing impoverishment (i.e. when payments push households below or further below the poverty line wherein the most basic standard of living is no longer ensured), result in financial hardship (Saksena et al., 2014). Whether health systems contribute to or alleviate poverty is dependent on coverage policies as well as a range of other factors, such as methods of provision and reimbursement. In this chapter we will focus on the impact of out-of-pocket health spending not only on those experiencing poverty, but also on those who are not necessarily impoverished but still experience financial hardship due to out-of-pocket spending.

This chapter explores the links between health systems and SDG1. While SDG3 is already dedicated to ensuring good health and monitoring progress towards universal health coverage, it is important to explicitly consider the spillover effects of the health system on poverty and financial hardship, particularly given the importance placed on poverty in the SDGs. This chapter will highlight the connection between Target 3.8, which addresses the need to achieve universal health coverage, and SDG1. In particular, the chapter will discuss SDG Indicator 3.8.2, which addresses the proportion of the population with high spending on health as a share of household financial resources. It argues that through coverage policy decisions, health systems play an important role in reducing poverty and financial hardship.

The next section of this chapter will briefly introduce SDG1 and its relevance to this chapter. The second section introduces common measures used to monitor financial hardship in health systems. Section three explores in greater detail how health systems – in particular, coverage policies – can affect the risk of poverty and financial hardship due to out-of-pocket payments. The fourth section presents two case studies:

- Latvia, where during the financial crisis in 2009 the government exempted people living in poverty or near poverty from copayments; and
- Germany, which in 2004 implemented copayments for outpatient care and lifted an income-based exemption.

These case studies demonstrate further the relative importance of copayment design and exemptions in reducing poverty.

5.2   Background

The title of SDG1 is very clear in its goal – No poverty – with an official objective to end poverty in all its forms everywhere. SDG1 is broken down further into a series of targets. Targets 1.1, 1.2, 1.3 and 1.B are the most relevant for this chapter. These targets describe an international commitment to:

- **1.1** by 2030, eradicate extreme poverty for all people everywhere, currently measured as people living on less than $1.25 a day;
- **1.2** by 2030, reduce at least by half the proportion of men, women and children of all ages living in poverty in all its dimensions according to national definitions;
- **1.3** implement nationally appropriate social protection systems and measures for all, including floors, and by 2030 achieve substantial coverage of the poor and the vulnerable; and
- **1.B** create sound policy frameworks at the national, regional and international levels, based on pro-poor and gender-sensitive development strategies, to support accelerated investment in poverty eradication actions.

In this chapter we will discuss how out-of-pocket health spending can cause individuals and households to experience financial hardship, to be at risk of impoverishment, to push them below poverty lines (including those in Targets 1.1 and 1.2), or further burden those who are already impoverished. Coverage policies are relevant to Target 1.3 as part of the social protection system for the poor and vulnerable, particularly mindful of how financial hardship intersects with illness. We shall see that health policy should be a leading consideration in new policy frameworks that attempt to eradicate poverty and improve incomes for

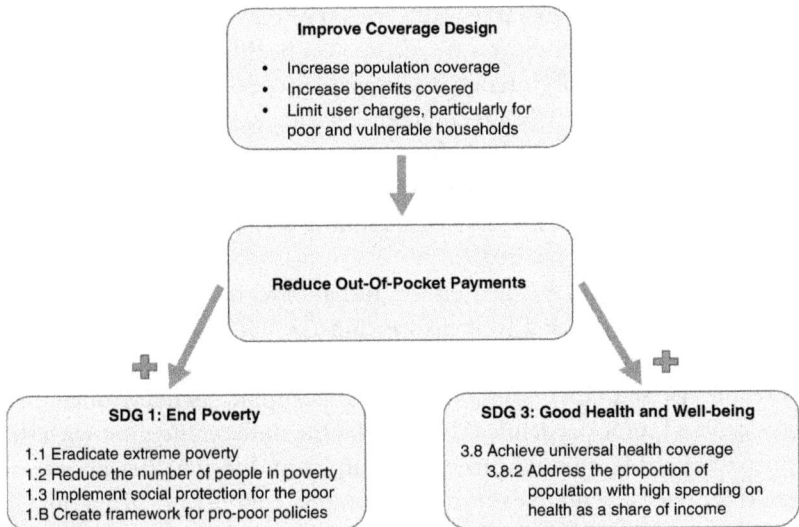

Fig. 5.1 Improvements to coverage design led to benefits for both SDG1 and SDG3

poor people in accordance with Target 1.B. Fig. 5.1 demonstrates how achieving progress in SDG Indicator 3.8.2 through improved coverage design has positive spillover effects on SDG1.

5.3 How can we measure the effects of out-of-pocket payments on financial hardship and poverty?

One of the main ways health systems influence the risk of financial hardship is through households' exposure to out-of-pocket payments. Out-of-pocket payments refer to user charges for covered health care goods and services, payments for non-covered goods and services, and informal payments. It excludes any pre-payment for health costs through public or private insurance.

A common way to measure the effect of out-of-pocket payments on the risk of financial hardship is by using two indicators: catastrophic and impoverishing expenditure incidence. These are commonly referred to under the umbrella term "financial protection indicators". Financial protection is monitored in the SDGs through Indicator 3.8.2. Indicator 3.8.2 is a type of catastrophic expenditure indicator: the proportion of the population spending large (10%) or very large (25%) shares of their total household expenditures or income on health.[1] This is one of the main indicators used globally to monitor progress towards universal health coverage. The UN's recommended data sources for monitoring financial protection are household budget surveys, usually conducted by national statistical offices. Household budget surveys record household spending on all goods and services, including on health, over a reporting period (United Nations, 2019).

While Indicator 3.8.2 is used for global SDG monitoring, there are numerous methods used to measure catastrophic spending incidence, all of which relate households' health expenditure to some measure of its resources and label households as catastrophic spenders once they have crossed some predefined threshold. One of the difficulties with the approach used by the indicator is that it is blind to whether poorer or wealthier people tend to exceed a certain percentage of their income in health spending, which can have significant consequences for the level of concern policymakers attribute to health spending (Wagstaff & van Doorslaer, 2003). In this chapter, we define the *incidence of catastrophic spending* based on the WHO Europe method, which is the share of households with out-of-pocket spending greater than 40% of household capacity to pay for care (Cylus, Thomson & Evetovits, 2018). The 40% share of household capacity to pay has been used in many studies of catastrophic spending, although with different definitions of capacity to pay (Wagstaff & van Doorslaer, 2003; Xu et al., 2007). Capacity to pay in the WHO Europe method is calculated by taking a household's total consumption expenditure and subtracting a normative amount that captures the costs of meeting basic needs for food, housing and utilities. This reflects a judgement that households must meet basic needs before having money available to pay for health care.

An important benefit of this approach is that the effective threshold for a household to become a catastrophic spender is lower for poor households, who must spend a higher proportion of their budget on

---

[1] There are also other methods for measuring financial protection that are not specifically mentioned in the SDGs. These include health spending as a proportion of income excluding actual food expenditure, health spending as a proportion of income excluding a standard amount representing subsistence food spending, and health spending as a proportion of income excluding subsistence-level spending on food, housing and utilities (Cylus, Thomson & Evetovits, 2018).

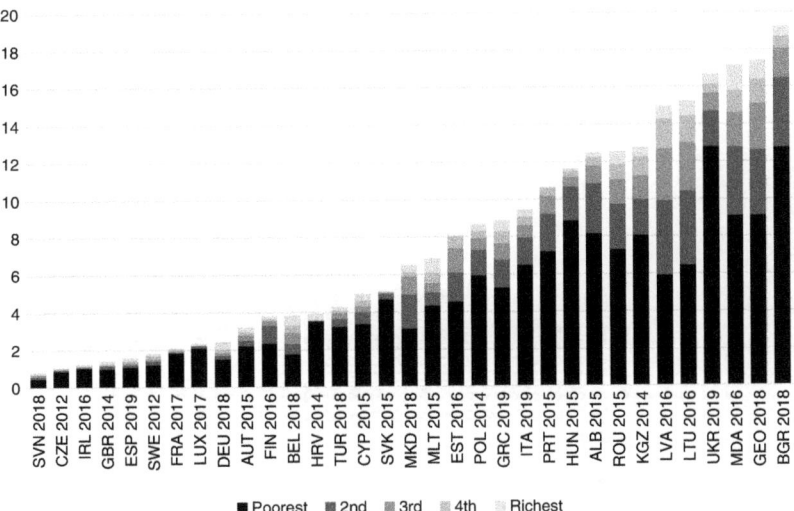

Fig. 5.2 Catastrophic spending using the WHO Europe method, latest year available

basic needs (and thus have a very limited capacity to pay for health), and higher for wealthier households. This creates a more progressive metric for measuring which groups of people suffer the most from high out-of-pocket spending. Fig. 5.2 shows that using the WHO Europe method of calculation, the poorest quintile of households experience the majority of the catastrophic health spending in most European countries.

Impoverishing expenditures are the other main financial protection indicator and perhaps the metric most directly relevant to SDG1. Households are defined as *impoverished* as a result of out-of-pocket health spending if their consumption before out-of-pocket spending was above a poverty line (or in the WHO Europe method, above the cost of meeting the aforementioned basic needs), and their spending after out-of-pocket costs was below the line. Households can also be considered *further impoverished* if their consumption before out-of-pocket spending was already below the poverty line or basic needs line and they still spent out-of-pocket for health care. As Fig. 5.3 shows, most of the burden of impoverishing spending in Europe falls on households that are already poor rather than those who are made poor by out-of-pocket spending. Households are also *at risk of impoverishment* under the WHO Europe method if their consumption after out-of-pocket spending

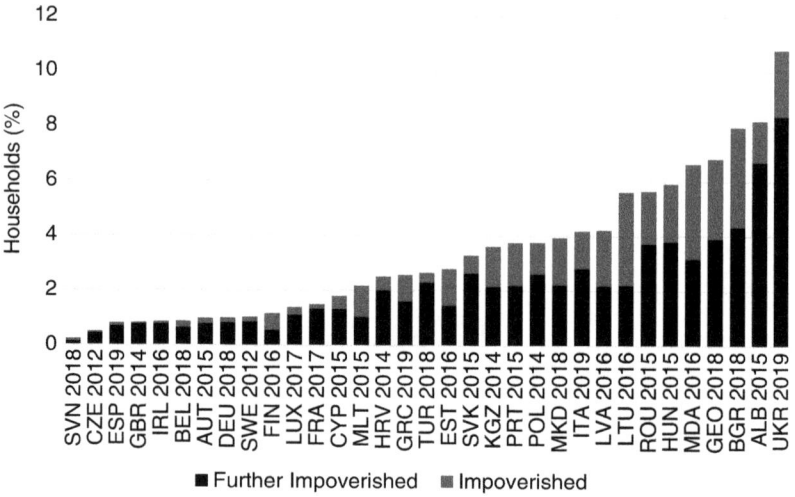

Fig. 5.3 Impoverishing spending by country, latest year available

is within 120% of the basic needs line (not shown in Fig. 5.3). The nuance in these metrics allows us to identify not just those who might fall below an internationally recognized consumption level, but also those who experience financial hardship without explicitly *becoming* poor according to binary indicators.

Catastrophic and impoverishing spending indicators on their own can be easily misinterpreted. For example, a country might have a low incidence of catastrophic spending not because care is affordable, but because large segments of the population face out-of-pocket costs that are beyond their means to pay. They may then use fewer services than needed, or no services at all. In this way, unmet need data gathered through self-reporting is an important complement to financial hardship measures.

5.4   How do health systems influence the risk of poverty and financial hardship?

Now that we have established indicators of financial hardship, we can say more about the links between out-of-pocket spending, catastrophic spending and impoverishment. How much a country relies on out-of-pocket payments to finance health care overall is a strong predictor of the incidence of catastrophic spending (Fig. 5.4). Catastrophic spending

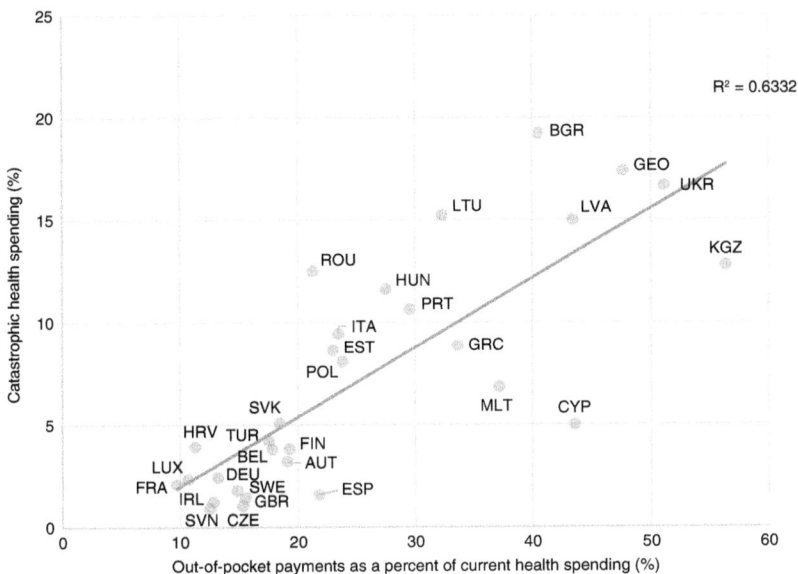

Fig. 5.4 Incidence of catastrophic health spending and out-of-pocket payments as a share of current spending on health, latest year available

tends to be much higher in countries where reliance on out-of-pocket spending to finance health care is high. Within Europe, Latvia, Lithuania and Hungary all have very elevated levels of catastrophic spending, each with more than 10% of their households experiencing catastrophic spending each year. All three countries rely on significantly higher levels of out-of-pocket spending to pay for health care than the OECD average (OECD, 2021). Fig. 5.5 also illustrates the positive correlation between a health system's reliance on out-of-pocket payments and impoverishing spending in European countries.

What then determines the level of out-of-pocket payments? Out-of-pocket payments for health care are partly determined by the level of public spending on health care (Fig. 5.6). The incidence of financial hardship due to out-of-pocket payments is more likely to be high when public spending on health is low in relation to gross domestic product *and* out-of-pocket payments account for a relatively high share of total spending on health (WHO & World Bank, 2019; Xu et al., 2007).

However, increases in public spending do not necessarily lead to reductions in out-of-pocket spending (WHO, 2019a). Mandating a

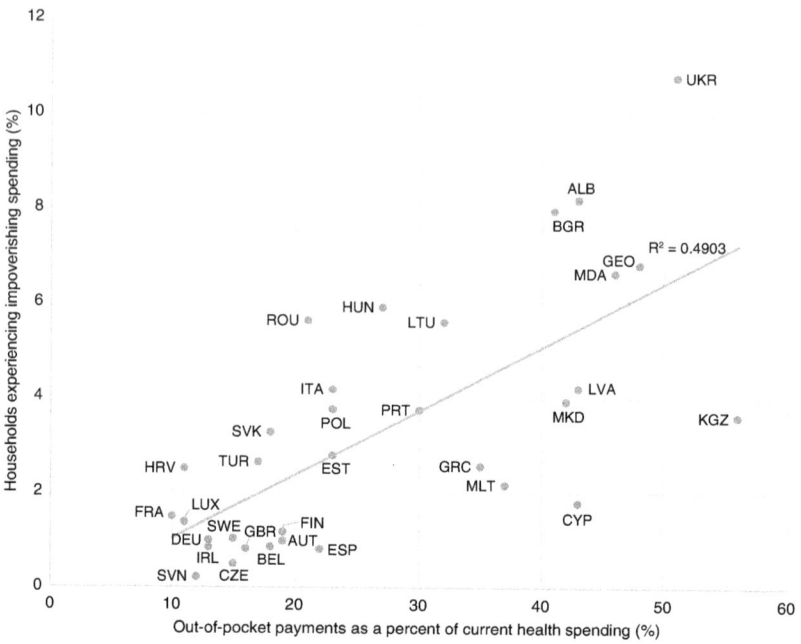

Fig. 5.5 Incidence of impoverishing (i.e., impoverished and further impoverished) spending and out-of-pocket payments as a share of current spending on health, latest year available

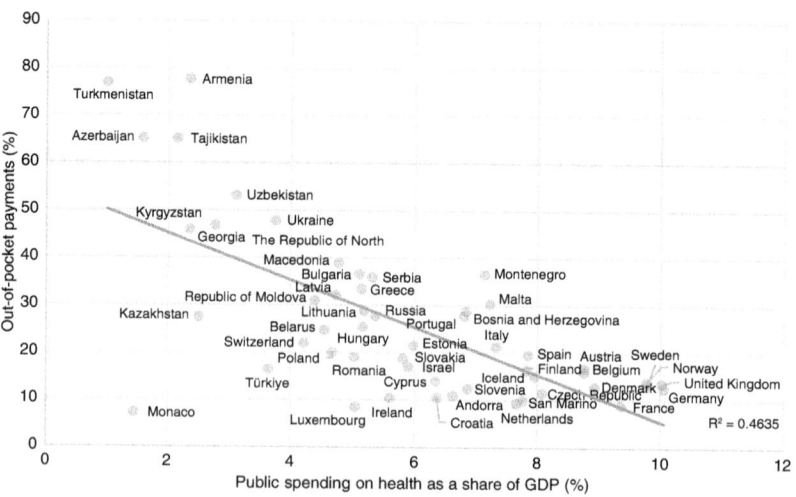

Fig. 5.6 Public spending on health as a share of GDP and out-of-pocket payments, WHO European Region, 2020

certain level of public spending on health has not been demonstrated to be an effective way to reduce out-of-pocket spending if not combined with other significant reforms to coverage policy design. For example, from 2004 to 2017 the government of Moldova committed to allocating 12% of its budget to health care every year, resulting in public spending on health that was significantly higher than the average lower-middle-income country in Europe (WHO, 2020). However, outpatient prescribed medicines were still subject to a percentage copayment of up to 50%. As a result, out-of-pocket spending grew over the period, as did the percent of households with catastrophic out-of-pocket spending (WHO, 2020). Indeed, many countries with similar levels of public spending on health differ in terms of their out-of-pocket spending. Public spending on health in 2019 accounted for 8% of GDP in both France and the United Kingdom, but while the former relied on out-of-pocket spending for 9% of health costs, the latter relied on it for 17% (WHO, 2022). Other aspects of health system design must account for the differences in out-of-pocket spending levels.

Coverage policy design is a crucial determinant of whether health systems contribute to or alleviate financial hardship. All health systems face budget constraints, which lead to rationing of care through coverage policy design. Budget constraints can lead to implicit rationing, such as gatekeeping and waiting times, as well as explicit rationing, such as coverage exclusions and out-of-pocket payments. This is true even in systems that purport to have achieved universal health coverage. We can conceptualize progress towards universal health coverage systems through an analysis of the coverage of people, services and cost. The goals of universal health coverage are most likely to be achieved when the entire population is covered, the right services are covered to meet the population's health needs, and costs are financed largely through pre-payment with risk pooling to avoid exposure to financial hardship or financial barriers when people need to access care. This is commonly described through the idea of the coverage cube, shown in Fig. 5.7.

Exploring the three dimensions of UHC helps to understand why countries might rely to a greater or lesser extent on out-of-pocket payments to pay for health care. We can use the conceptualization of the coverage cube as a series of tradeoffs to show how allocating limited resources towards each of the three dimensions affects out-of-pocket payments in different ways (Ochalek, Manthalu & Smith, 2020).

The first dimension is the level of population coverage. Many systems exclude individuals from the health system based on employment,

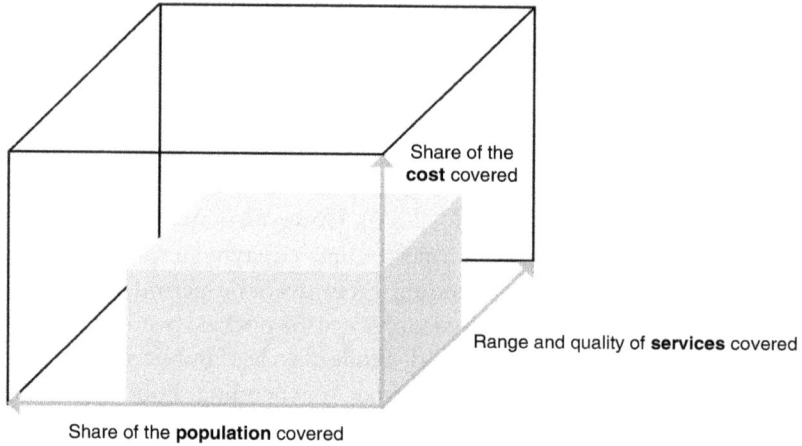

Share of the **population** covered

Fig. 5.7 The coverage cube demonstrates the three dimensions of health coverage

citizenship, age or income. In some countries, publicly funded services are restricted only to a certain segment of the population, for example, dental care for adults in the English NHS. This means that excluded patients must pay privately if they need care. Population entitlement to publicly financed health care is a prerequisite for protection from financial hardship but does not guarantee it. The share of population entitled is not an intrinsically good indicator of exposure to financial hardship. Incidence of catastrophic health spending in European countries with 100% population coverage varies significantly, from 1% to 14% of households (WHO, 2019b). Reviews of health insurance reforms in nine developing countries found that expanded population coverage was linked to decreased out-of-pocket expenses in six of the countries, but to an increase in out-of-pocket expenses in three of them, partly because of increased service utilization due to coverage (Lagomarsino et al., 2012; Wagstaff & Lindelow, 2008). In some countries, entitlement to care is linked to employment; this can lead to those in precarious or unstable working conditions being excluded from coverage. European countries that have linked health coverage to employment, such as Greece, saw a rise in catastrophic health spending among middle-class households and a rise in unmet health need among those with lower incomes in the years following the Great Recession, when unemployment rose dramatically and many people lost health care coverage (WHO, 2019b).

The second dimension considers the breadth of the benefits package as well as volume limits for treatments that are covered by statutory health care coverage, which can result in long waiting times. If the benefits package is narrow or there are long waiting times, those who can afford it may pay out-of-pocket for care, contributing to poverty and financial hardship. There is considerable variability in the types of goods and services countries cover (WHO, 2019b). Although Health Technology Assessment agencies exist in many high-income health systems to investigate the cost-effectiveness of covering a certain medical intervention, the majority do not make binding decisions and in most cases it is not clear that their recommendations are considered in coverage decisions (Fontrier, Visintin & Kanavos, 2021). Service restrictions can also occur when people are promised benefits that are not supported by adequate funding. This can result in implicit rationing of care through informal payments, which is a significant problem in several European countries. Countries with higher levels of informal payments for health care tend to have higher rates of catastrophic spending (WHO, 2019b). Even when not the primary cause of health-related financial hardship in a country overall, informal payments make it impossible for governments to protect poor people from high out-of-pocket costs through means-tested exemptions. The highly unpredictable nature of informal payments also abrogates the consumption-smoothing benefits to health insurance, either voluntary or public.

The third, and most important, mechanism by which out-of-pocket payments lead to financial hardship is through user charges. While all European countries have some form of user charges, the systems with the strongest financial protection either apply them sparingly or make efforts to protect against financial hardship. Three of the most relevant copayment policy mechanisms are using fixed copayments rather than percentage-based coinsurance, user charge exemptions for poor people, and out-of-pocket maximums (i.e. caps).

Fixed copayments are a pre-set amount that a user pays that are not dependent on the items' list price. Percentage-based coinsurance refers to a system in which patients will pay for a certain percentage of the list price of an item. The countries that use percentage-based coinsurance tend to have higher rates of catastrophic health spending than countries with low fixed copayments (WHO, 2019b). Poland and Slovakia, for example, have similar out-of-pocket spending as a share of current health expenditure and similar poverty rates (Thomson, Cylus & Evetovits, 2019), but the rate of catastrophic health spending in the former is more than twice as high than that in the latter (WHO, 2019b). One difference is that Poland uses percentage-based coinsurance while Slovakia uses fixed copayments for user charges associated with outpatient medicines. Percentage-based coinsurance shifts financial risks from the health system to the patient, which in effect creates a regressive cost policy for the poorest users of health services. Percentage-based coinsurance also exposes patients to high levels of price uncertainty, especially when prices are not known to the patient in advance.

Another set of copayment policy options that have proven particularly effective in limiting financial hardship are user charge exemptions for poor people. This is especially the case for those who are impoverished and unable to meet their basic needs even before spending out-of-pocket on health. In Germany, the switch from user charge exemptions for poor people to an annual cap on copayments led to an increase in catastrophic spending, particularly among the poorest consumption quintile (WHO, 2019b). In Latvia, the end of exemptions from copayments for poor people led to a similarly sharp rise in catastrophic spending in the poorest quintile (WHO, 2018a). We will cover these examples in more detail in our case studies.

The justification for user charges for universal health care systems includes additional revenue raising for the health system and reduction of potentially inappropriate demand (i.e. moral hazard) (King's Fund, 2005). However, a number of counterarguments to these justifications have developed. In order for insurance to lead to inappropriate demand, provider incentives must be aligned with overtreatment and consumers must have a significant influence over their treatment choice. This may be true in systems with widespread use of fee-for-service reimbursement but is unlikely to occur in systems that use capitation, fixed salaries or pay-for-performance. Supply constraints, such as direct rationing, waiting times, gatekeeping and payer prior authorization, are often used to deal with potential moral hazard even in systems that have user charges. There is also consistent evidence that user charges reduce medically necessary and unnecessary care equally, which can have negative effects on population health (Thomson, Foubiser & Mossialos, 2010; WHO, 2019b). Out-of-pocket user charges for certain prescription drugs and preventative treatments in the UK, for example, were found to be not efficient as they increased long-term health costs to the NHS (King's Fund, 2005). Fixed charges not related to ability to pay disproportionately lower access to care for the poor, raising issues of equity.

Furthermore, institutions such as the NHS have not traditionally asserted clear boundaries between the basic package of care and supplemental health services (King's Fund, 2005).

It is also worth reviewing the evidence on whether encouraging individuals to take matters into their own hands by purchasing complementary health insurance would be a good way to reduce catastrophic spending. While there are a few countries where complementary health insurance covers out-of-pocket payments (such as Slovenia, France and Croatia), this is the exception rather than the norm. More often complementary health insurance is used in a limited capacity by those who can afford to pay for it to obtain preferential access to care, rather than to provide financial protection. In the European context, research suggests that expanded use of complementary insurance is not an effective solution to lack of population coverage, restrictions in the benefits package, or widespread user charges, with no strong correlation between complementary insurance levels and out-of-pocket costs (WHO, 2019b). Moreover, complementary insurance adds a layer of complexity to coverage reform and individual health management to address issues that could also be solved through changes to the main coverage. Only reform to the design of coverage policies has been shown to reduce out-of-pocket costs, and thus limit financial burdens on households.

5.5 Country case studies

To better understand how health systems and coverage policy influence the risk of poverty and financial hardship, we present two case studies: Latvia and Germany. These cases will demonstrate the co-benefits between improving health systems and decreasing financial hardship that we have discussed in a real-world environment.

5.5.1 Case 1: Latvia

To cope with the hardship caused by the recession of 2008, Latvian government ministries working in collaboration with external stakeholders improved financial protection for the poorest segments of the population through temporary user charge exemptions. In 2012, however, Latvia discontinued this exemption from copayments for all but the very poorest individuals; the end of exemptions led to an increase in financial hardship for poor people.

All Latvian citizens, as well as many immigrant groups, are guaranteed access to health care under the Latvian National Health Service (NHS). The opportunity for out-of-pocket spending derives primarily from a relatively narrow benefits package and user charges rather than explicit population exclusion from coverage.

In 2009, Latvia raised copayments across almost all services as part of fiscal restraints required by external lenders during the Great Recession. After the financial crisis that arose as a result of the 2008 recession, the Latvian government agreed to cuts to public sector expenditure, tax increases, and public administration reforms, collectively known as the Economic Stabilization and Growth Revival Programme (Taube, Mitenbergs & Sagan, 2015). The lenders included the International Monetary Fund (IMF), the EU and the World Bank, which also provided technical support. The Latvian Cabinet of Ministers explicitly mentioned health care spending as one of the sectors to which public sector cuts would be made, giving the Ministry of Health the space to implement a copayment rise (Taube, Mitenbergs & Sagan, 2015). Some of these increases were considerable – the daily copayment for inpatient hospital stays more than doubled. At the same time, Latvia also introduced the Social Safety Net strategy in 2009, granting exemptions from those user charges for households with incomes below €171 per person per month and substantial reductions to those with incomes below €213. The Social Safety Net strategy was financially supported by the external lenders as a way to mitigate the worst adverse effects of the recession on poorer households. In this sense, changes to the design of the health system were used to create co-benefits for the public sector financial position and for financial hardship.

The health reforms during the financial crisis, including the low-income copayment exemptions, took place with few consultations with domestic health system stakeholders (Taube, Mitenbergs & Sagan, 2015). The driving force was a collaboration between government ministries and external lenders. Table 5.1 shows the governance tools used and actions taken during the 2009 health reforms and Social Safety Net strategy. Overall, the reforms were supported by the most important governmental stakeholders, the Ministry of Finance and the Cabinet, giving the Ministry of Health the leeway to implement the copayment rise and low-income exemption with little conflict. As summarized in Table 5.2, the issue also had high political importance given its relevance to the reforms required by the external lenders. Due

Table 5.1 *Possible governance actions to achieve SDG1 in Latvia*

			Possible governance actions with these tools								
			Goals and targets	Evidence support	Policy guidance	Implementation and management	Coordination	Advocacy	Monitoring and evaluation	Financial support	Legal mandate
Tools	Plan	Plan	x		x			x		x	x
	Indicators and Targets	Indicators	x		x				x		
		Targets									
	Budgeting	Pooled budget									
		Shared objectives	x		x	x	x	x		x	
		Coordinated budgeting				x	x	x		x	
	Organization	Ministerial linkages	x					x		x	
		Specific ministers							x		
		Organization	x			x		x		x	
		Legislative committees									
		Interdepartmental committees/units									
		Departmental mergers									
		Civic engagement									
	Accountability	Transparent data	x			x		x	x	x	
		Regular reporting	x			x		x	x	x	
		Independent agency/evaluators	x						x	x	
		Support for civil society									
		Legal rights									

Table 5.2 *Political importance and conflict: eliminating poverty in Latvia*

		Conflict	
		Low	High
Political	High	x	
importance	Low		

to the overall burden of the recession and copayment rise on the poor in Latvia, policies to alleviate financial hardship also had intrinsically high political importance.

The 2009 exemption that the Latvian government put into place with support from external lenders was effective at mitigating the contribution of health spending to financial hardship. The share of households in the poorest quintile reporting no out-of-pocket spending improved from 58% to 70% from 2008 to 2010 (WHO, 2018a). Over the same period, the rate of catastrophic spending for the poorest quintile declined even while overall catastrophic spending in Latvia increased, likely due to the combined effects of the copayment rise and income-based exemptions (WHO, 2018a).

However, the low-income exemption policy was pared back in 2012 after the World Bank ended financial and technical support, leaving the policy's continuation by the Latvian government financially untenable. Only those with incomes below €128 per person per month were still eligible for any reduction, exposing many low-income people to user charges. The effects on financial hardship for the poor were significant. Among the lowest income quintile, the share of households reporting no out-of-pocket payments declined from 70% in 2010 to 57% in 2013 (WHO, 2018a). The rate of catastrophic spending for the poorest households increased significantly, and by 2016, 15% of Latvian households experienced catastrophic health spending – among the highest rates in the EU (OECD, 2021; WHO, 2018a). Inpatient hospital admissions also declined significantly from 2012 to 2013, reversing a longstanding trend and implying that much of the reduction was from unmet need due to unaffordable health costs (WHO, 2018a).

The Social Safety Net strategy was successful at reducing health costs as a source of financial hardship from 2009 to 2012. Without collaboration between the external lenders and the relevant Latvian ministries, it would have been significantly more difficult for the Latvian government to put financial resources towards the Social Safety Net strategy during a period of fiscal restraint, particularly when the rest of the population was subject to a copayment rise. Indeed, once intersectoral support for the policy in the form of World Bank assistance was withdrawn, the Latvian government was unable to continue the most important provisions of the policy on its own despite the clear benefits for financial protection.

5.5.2   Case 2: Germany

Overall financial protection in Germany is strong, in line with many other European countries with low reliance on out-of-pocket spending and high public spending on health. Population coverage is near universal, as health insurance has been mandatory for the entire population since 2009. However, Germany's experiences over the past two decades show that coverage policy decisions have notable effects on the risk of financial hardship.

Germany introduced copayments for outpatient visits in 2004 as part of the Hartz reforms, which were aimed at reducing public spending. At the same time, Germany shifted from fixed copayments to percentage-based coinsurance for outpatient medicines and abolished exemptions from user charges for low-income people. These changes shifted some financial responsibility for care to households, coinciding with an increase in the share of out-of-pocket spending on outpatient care from 6.4% in 2003 to 13.8% in 2008. This increase was even more pronounced among the poorest quintile, leading to implications for financial protection. The share of the poorest quintile of households with catastrophic out-of-pocket payments in Germany more than doubled from 2003 to 2008 (WHO, 2018b). The share at risk of impoverishment, impoverished or further impoverished after out-of-pocket payments rose from around 2% to almost 6% (WHO, 2018b).

In 2012, an intersectoral consensus of providers, patients and parliamentarians led to the abolition of copayments for outpatient visits, although the percentage-based coinsurance for outpatient medicines remained and the low-income exemptions were not reinstated. From 2008 to 2013, the share of out-of-pocket spending on outpatient care fell from 13.8% to 6.5%. By 2013, the share of the poorest quintile experiencing catastrophic spending had fallen from 2008 levels but remained above the pre-2004 level (WHO, 2018b). The share of households at risk of impoverishment, impoverished or further impoverished after out-of-pocket payments fell to around 4%, which, while an improvement from 2008, was still twice as high as pre-2004. The fact that the incidence of households impoverished due to health costs remained higher than pre-2004 suggests income-based exemptions from out-of-pocket payments had been effective at providing financial protection.

The decision to abolish copayments for outpatient visits was made through a unanimous vote of the German Federal Parliament following intersectoral collaboration between parliamentarians of multiple parties, the health minister, and civil society groups representing providers and patients (Table 5.3). The copayment was seen by parliamentarians as providing insufficient revenue for the administrative costs it necessitated (Olm et al., 2020). It was largely opposed by providers, who felt burdened by the effort of administering the copayment, as well as patients (Kilham, 2015). The issue was given high levels of coverage by the German media, amplifying its political importance (Olm et al., 2020).

Table 5.3 *Possible governance actions to achieve SDG1 in Germany*

Tools			Goals and targets	Evidence support	Policy guidance	Implementation and management	Coordination	Advocacy	Monitoring and evaluation	Financial support	Legal mandate
	Plan	Plan	x	x	x	x	x	x			x
	Indicators and targets	Indicators	x	x					x	x	
		Targets	x	x					x	x	
	Budgeting	Pooled budget									
		Shared objectives									
		Coordinated budgeting									

Table 5.3 *(Cont.)*

			Possible governance actions with these tools								
Tools	**Organization**	Ministerial linkages									
		Specific ministers	x	x	x	x	x	x		x	x
		Organization	x				x	x			
		Legislative committees									
		Interdepartmental committees/units									
		Departmental mergers									
		Civic engagement	x	x	x			x			
	Accountability	Transparent data		x	x			x	x		
		Regular reporting		x	x			x	x		
		Independent agency/evaluators									
		Support for civil society	x	x	x			x			
		Legal rights									

Table 5.4 *Political importance and conflict: eliminating poverty in Germany*

		Conflict	
		Low	**High**
Political importance	High	x	
	Low		

Given the convergence of interests in abolishing the copayment – federal government, providers and patients – and the widespread nature of the administrative burden, we can categorize the decision as being of high political importance (Table 5.4). The political conflict, in contrast, can be categorized as low as there was widespread consensus for the measure throughout the German Federal Parliament. The key to the success of this change was intersectoral collaboration between parliamentarians, patients and providers. The co-benefits of collaboration are illustrated by the reduction in financial hardship on the population at large as well as the increased access to outpatient care and lower administrative costs on providers.

5.6 Conclusion

The goal of policymakers should be to create policies that ensure that people who are financially vulnerable are not exposed to further hardship as a result of using health services. This goal will be most effectively achieved through intersectoral collaboration between stakeholders with expertise in public finance and health, who can work together to pass policies that will improve the health system while decreasing financial hardship. While not explicitly included in SDG1, people who face potential financial hardship from out-of-pocket health spending should be prioritized through health system policies along with those who face explicit impoverishment. To reduce both poverty and financial hardship in the context of limited public resources, it is advisable, despite the marginal political support, to enact policies that benefit the most disadvantaged households. To ensure these policies are effective, policymakers must have the ability to identify health services that lead to financial hardship and the people most affected by them. While increasing public investment in health overall is a first step, many countries will need to reconsider coverage policies to improve financial hardship outcomes.

Specifically, countries should ensure full population coverage, a comprehensive benefits package, and limited user charges, both for the sake of improving health outcomes as well as to help eradicate poverty. For user charge policy in particular, the countries that have had the most success have implemented policies including fixed copayments rather than percentage-based coinsurance, user charge exemptions for poor households, and out-of-pocket maximums. Of the three, especially in the context of poverty eradication, means-tested exemptions from user charges are likely most effective, though there can be administrative, logistical and measurement challenges in means-testing, in part due to a lack of information about household financial resources in real-time.

The threat from ineffective coverage policy that fails to adequately protect people from financial hardship and impoverishment is clear.

Policies that shift financial responsibility for care onto patients through higher out-of-pocket costs, such as those in the Germany and Latvia case studies, have led to an increase in catastrophic health expenditures. Expanded population coverage alone does not protect individuals from financial hardship, as a full 9% of people in the United States with employer-sponsored health insurance (ESHI) have declared bankruptcy due to medical costs (KFF, 2019). Poorly designed coverage policy has led to the sickest patients simultaneously suffering from disease and the threat of ruinous costs. If countries wish to make progress on reducing poverty and financial hardship, they should focus coverage design efforts on reducing the financial burden placed on those who are most vulnerable.

References

Cylus J, Thomson S, Evetovits T (2018). Catastrophic health spending in Europe: equity and policy implications of different calculation methods. Bull World Health Organ, 96:599–609. (http://dx.doi.org/10.2471/BLT.18.209031)

Fontrier A, Visintin E, Kanavos P (2021). Similarities and Differences in Health Technology Assessment Systems and Implications for Coverage Decisions: Evidence from 32 Countries. Pharmacoecon Open, 6(3):315–328. (https://doi.org/10.1007/s41669-021-00311-5)

KFF (2019). Kaiser Family Foundation/LA Times Survey of Adults with Employer-Sponsored Health Insurance. The Henry J. Kaiser Family Foundation. (https://files.kff.org/attachment/Report-KFF-LA-Times-Survey-of-Adults-with-Employer-Sponsored-Health-Insurance)

Kilham R (2015). Is national health spending on an unaffordable trajectory? Clin Exp Optom, 98(2):105–106. (https://doi-org.proxy.lib.umich.edu/10.1111/cxo.12245)

King's Fund (2005). Co-payments and charges in the NHS. (https://www.kingsfund.org.uk/sites/default/files/field/field_publication_file/Consultation-response-co-payments-charges-dec-2005.pdf)

Lagomarsino G, Garabrant A, Adyas A et al. (2012). Moving towards universal health coverage: health insurance reforms in nine developing countries in Africa and Asia. Lancet, 380(9845):933–943. (https://www-sciencedirect-com.proxy.lib.umich.edu/science/article/pii/S0140673612611477)

Ochalek J, Manthalu G, Smith P (2020). Squaring the cube: Towards an operational model of optimal universal health coverage. J Health Econ, 70:102282. (https://www.sciencedirect.com/science/article/pii/S0167629619301560)

OECD (2021). Financial hardship and out-of-pocket expenditure. OECD iLibrary. (https://www.oecd-ilibrary.org/sites/ae3016b9-en/1/3/5/4/index .html?itemId=/content/publication/ae3016b9-en&_csp_=ca413da5d44587 bc56446341952c275e&itemIGO=oecd&itemContentType=book)

Olm M, Donnachie E, Tauscher M et al. (2020). Impact of the abolition of copayments on the GP-centred coordination of care in Bavaria, Germany: analysis of routinely collected claims data. BMJ Open, 10(9):e035575. (https://www.ncbi.nlm.nih.gov/pmc/articles/PMC7470646/)

Ravallion M (2010). Poverty Lines across the World. The World Bank, Development Research Group. Policy Research Working Paper 5284. (https://documents1.worldbank.org/curated/en/298951468174919253/ pdf/WPS5284.pdf)

Saksena P, Hsu J, Evans D (2014). Financial Risk Protection and Universal Health Coverage: Evidence and Measurement Challenges. PLOS Med, 11(9). (https://www.ncbi.nlm.nih.gov/pmc/articles/PMC4171370/)

Taube M, Mitenbergs U, Sagan A (2015). The impact of the crisis on the health system and health in Latvia. In: Maresso A, Mladovsky P, Thomson S et al. (eds) Economic crisis, health systems and health in Europe. Copenhagen: European Observatory on Health Systems and Policies. (https://www.ncbi .nlm.nih.gov/books/NBK447888/)

Thomson S, Cylus J, Evetovits T (2019). Can people afford to pay for health care? New evidence on financial protection in Europe. Eurohealth 25(3):41–46.

Thomson S, Foubiser T, Mossialos E (2010). Can user charges make health care more efficient? BMJ, 341:487–489. (https://www.bmj.com/content/ bmj/341/7771/Analysis.full.pdf)

United Nations (2019). SDG indicator metadata: Indicator 3.8.2. UN Statistics Division. (https://unstats.un.org/sdgs/metadata/files/Metadata-03-08-02. pdf)

United Nations (2022). Goal 1: End poverty in all its forms everywhere. UN Statistics Division. (https://unstats.un.org/sdgs/report/2016/goal-01/)

Wagstaff A, van Doorslaer E (2003). Catastrophe and impoverishment in paying for health care: with applications to Vietnam 1993–1998. J Health Econ, 12(11):921–933. (https://onlinelibrary-wiley-com.proxy.lib.umich .edu/doi/pdf/10.1002/hec.776)

Wagstaff A, Lindelow M (2008). Can insurance increase financial risk? The curious case of health insurance in China. J Health Econ, 27(4):990–1005. (https://doi-org.proxy.lib.umich.edu/10.1016/j.jhealeco.2008.02.002)

WHO (2018a). Can people afford to pay for health care? New evidence on financial protection in Latvia. (https://www.euro.who.int/__data/assets/ pdf_file/0008/373580/Can-people-afford-to-payLatvia-WHO-FP-006.pdf)

WHO (2018b). Can people afford to pay for health care? New evidence on financial protection in Germany. (https://www.euro.who.int/__data/assets/pdf_file/0004/373585/Can-people-afford-to-payGermany-WHO-FP-008-4.pdf)

WHO (2019a). Global spending on health: a world in transition. License: CC BY-NC-SA 3.0 IGO. (https://www.who.int/publications/i/item/WHO-HIS-HGF-HFWorkingPaper-19.4)

WHO (2019b). Can people afford to pay for health care? New evidence on financial protection in Europe. (https://apps.who.int/iris/bitstream/handle/10665/311654/9789289054058-eng.pdf?sequence=1&isAllowed=y)

WHO (2020). Can people afford to pay for health care? New evidence on financial protection in the Republic of Moldova. (https://apps.who.int/iris/bitstream/handle/10665/331667/9789289054959-eng.pdf)

WHO (2022). Global Health Expenditure Database [online database]. (https://apps.who.int/nha/database/ViewData/Indicators/en)

WHO, World Bank (2019). Global Monitoring Report on Financial Protection in Health 2019. (https://www.who.int/healthinfo/universal_health_coverage/report/fp_gmr_2019.pdf)

World Bank (2021). Universal Health Coverage. Understanding Poverty. (https://www.worldbank.org/en/topic/universalhealthcoverage-1)

Xu, Ke, et al. "Protecting households from catastrophic health spending." Health affairs 26.4 (2007): 972–983.

6 | SDG4, education: education as a lever for sustainable development

KRISTINE SØRENSEN

6.1 Introduction

During the past generations, education has become a principal pathway to good health, financial security, stable employment and social success. The remarkable progress reaffirms the belief that education is one of the most powerful and proven leverages for sustainable development and peace. Education is strongly associated with life expectancy, morbidity and health behaviours, and educational attainment plays an important role in health by shaping opportunities, employment and income. As such, it is widely recognized that health and education are mutually influential. Education can create opportunities for better health, and an individual's health can influence their educational achievement and outcomes. However, the provision of quality schools, textbooks and teachers can result in effective education only if a child or student is in school and ready and able to learn. A child who is hungry or sick will not be able to complete a basic education of good quality. The challenge remains on how to develop and sustain empowered learners who can benefit from health to develop their potential and lifelong learning opportunities.

The vision of the 2030 Agenda for Sustainable Development envisages a world with universal literacy and with equitable and universal access to quality education at all levels (United Nations, 2015). The ambitions regarding education are essentially captured in the Sustainable Development Goal 4 (SDG4) of the 2030 Agenda which aims to "ensure inclusive and equitable quality education and promote lifelong learning opportunities for all" by 2030. The targets include free, equitable and quality education; access to early childhood development; and safe, healthy and inclusive schools (United Nations, 2015). Coordinated by UNESCO, *The Education 2030 Framework for Action* which was adopted in 2015 provides a framework for action through partnerships, policy guidance, capacity development, monitoring and advocacy (UNESCO, 2021). Nevertheless, according to UNESCO, every goal in the 2030 Agenda requires education to empower people with the knowledge, skills and values to live in dignity, build their lives and contribute to their societies.

Mostly, educational attainment is treated as a driver of opportunities in adulthood; however, education also functions to reproduce inequality across generations. The recognition of the dual impact of education is critical to developing education policies that would avoid unintended consequences of increasing inequalities. Moreover, education and health are inextricably embedded in different historical and social contexts which may induce substantial variations in health-education associations that need to be acknowledged to exacerbate or reduce educational disparities in health (Zajacova & Lawrence, 2018).

While governments hold the main responsibility for ensuring the right to quality education, the 2030 Agenda is a universal and collective commitment. It requires political will, global and regional collaboration and the engagement of all governments, civil society, the private sector, youth, United Nations and other multilateral agencies to tackle educational challenges and build systems that are inclusive, equitable and relevant to all learners for the benefit of social development and sustainability (UNESCO, 2021).

Education as a social determinant of health has been widely explored and much evidence is available (Ross & Wu, 1995). Population groups defined by a low educational status consistently show a greater disparity in terms of health despite differences between and within countries (Gumà, Solé-Auró & Arpino, 2019). Moreover, education influences an individual's health at different life-course stages (from adulthood to advanced age), as well as mediates the long-term influence of early-life conditions on health (Arpino, Gumà & Julià, 2018). The impact of education on health differs between women and men (Gumà, Solé-Auró & Arpino, 2019) and, as a consequence, both lowers female representation in the labour market and reinforces the gender wage gap (Ross & Mirowsky, 2010; Ross, Masters & Hummer, 2012). Nevertheless, the role of health on education and its contribution to social sustainability is less prominent. Therefore, the aim of this chapter is to explore the co-benefits of health on education as a lever of the sustainable development goals. Research and transformative health actions are showcased with regards to health literacy, school health programmes, and health-related workforce capacity to reveal how health becomes an enabler and a proponent for progress on education and sustainable development.

6.2 Background

The 2030 Agenda for Sustainable Development is a plan of action with 17 goals for people, planet and prosperity. SDG4 on education aims to ensure inclusive and equitable quality education and promote lifelong learning opportunities for all by ensuring that all children complete free, equitable and quality primary, secondary and tertiary education leading to relevant and effective learning outcomes. Moreover, SDG4 helps to increase the number of youth and adults who have relevant skills for employment, decent jobs and entrepreneurship to promote sustainable development, and ensures the relevant workforce conduct education without leaving anyone behind (United Nations, 2015).

Generally, basic literacy skills across the world have improved tremendously. According to the *SDG Tracker*, so far major progress has been made towards increasing access to education at all levels, particularly for women and girls. The total enrolment rate in developing regions reached more than 90% in 2015 and the number of children out of school dropped by almost half (SDG-Tracker.org). Yet bolder efforts are needed to achieve universal educational goals for all. According to UNESCO, to create a more sustainable world and to engage with issues related to sustainability, individuals must acquire knowledge, skills, values and attitudes that empower them to contribute to sustainable development as change-makers. Empowered learners are enabled to take informed decisions and act responsibly for environmental integrity, economic viability and a just society, for present and future generations (UNESCO, 2017).

6.3 Education as a structural determinant of health

The level of educational attainment is increasingly being recognized as an important social determinant of health (CSDH, 2008). While higher educational attainment can play a significant role in shaping employment opportunities, it can also increase the capacity for better decisionmaking regarding one's health and provide scope for increasing social and personal resources that are vital for physical and mental health.

People who have access to quality education throughout their lives tend to stay healthier than people without access to quality education. Not only does education give individuals a chance at upward mobility, which places them in better financial circumstances to access quality health care, it also keeps them better informed about how to take care of their health. Less education is linked to lower income, which is linked to poorer health. Numerous studies show that people in lower socioeconomic situations experience more obesity, asthma, diabetes, heart disease and other health problems than people in better financial circumstances. Moreover, higher education helps people secure higher paying work with fewer safety risks. Ultimately, more highly educated people have greater economic resources to afford things like better housing far away from environmental toxins and expert doctors trained in the most effective techniques.

Essentially, improved health and educational outcomes in school increase the potential for greater economic benefits for children when they reach adulthood because of enhanced career opportunities as well as better physical and emotional health, and these effects can be passed down to future generations (McDaid, 2016).

6.4   Health as a proponent of education

Evidently, health is also a proponent of education, and it will be explored in more detail using three concrete examples. First, the rising discourse of health literacy is presented and contextualized with regards to its impact on educational outcomes. Second, the role of learning for health and wellbeing in school settings is highlighted as a systemic approach to amplify the mutual impact of health and education. Lastly, the important role of the health workforce as an educational capacity is discussed as an instrument to lever societal impact on sustainable development.

6.4.1   *Health literacy*

Health literacy entails the knowledge, motivation and competencies to access, understand, appraise and apply information to form judgements and make decisions regarding healthcare, disease prevention and health promotion in everyday life to maintain and improve quality of life during the life course (Sørensen et al., 2012). Increasingly, the importance of pushing the health literacy agenda forward is being recognized by decisionmakers (Quaglio et al., 2017). Strategies and means are being applied to bridge the gap, for instance, through the implementation of national action plans on health literacy and intervention programmes (Rowlands et al., 2018).

Health literacy can be measured at individual, family, organizational, community, population and societal levels (WHO, 2013). The
first European Health Literacy Survey found that on average almost
one in two of the surveyed adult population had suboptimal general
health literacy and that this finding was linked to lower self-rated
health, higher rates of chronic (i.e. long-term) health conditions, more
adverse lifestyle choices (exercise, body mass index and alcohol) and
higher use of health services (Sørensen et al., 2015). Despite the efforts
of many European welfare states to develop effective healthcare systems
and educational systems, limited health literacy remains a challenge for
certain population groups such as people of age, people facing socioeconomic deprivation or those impacted by ethnic minority-related
stigma (M-POHL, 2021).

Within the WHO European Region, health literacy is recognized
as an enabling measure to advance the implementation of the 2030
agenda by strengthening leadership and governance, reducing health
inequalities, preventing disease, establishing healthy settings and achieving universal health coverage, and to achieve the highest attainable

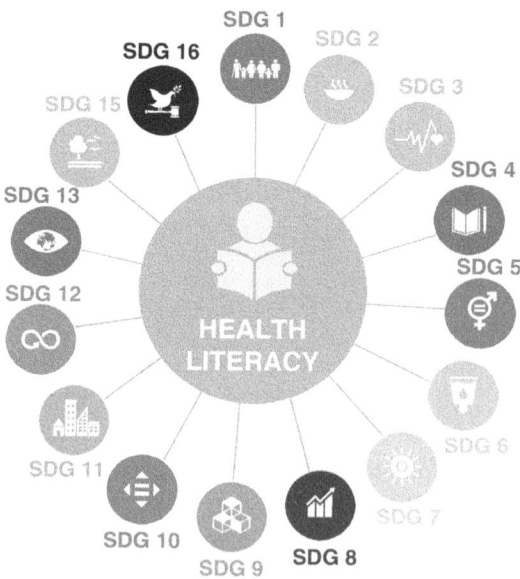

Fig. 6.1 SDGs influenced by strengthening health literacy

Source: WHO, 2021

standard of health and wellbeing for all at all ages and for future generations (WHO, 2019). Health literacy accelerates the outcomes of various SDGs in various ways (WHO, 2021).

6.4.2   *The impact of health literacy on educational outcomes*

Health literacy impacts educational outcomes, directly and indirectly (Dadaczynski et al., 2020; McDaid, 2016; Sørensen & Okan, 2020). The indirect path is demonstrated by the well established causal influence health indicators can have on different educational aspects such as school grades, early school-leaving or school attendance (Dadaczynski, 2012). Students who have higher levels of health literacy perceive their health to be better than those who perceive their health literacy to be lower (Paakkari et al., 2020). Similarly, they report having better self-esteem, being more satisfied with their life, having fewer health complaints (for example, psychosomatic complaints), and they also have more health knowledge (Paakkari et al., 2019). Better health literacy has also been associated with a lesser likelihood of becoming over- or underweight, as well as with several positive health behaviours, such as increased level of physical activity (Shih et al., 2016), less use of alcohol and less smoking (Fleary, Joseph & Pappagianopoulos, 2018), and better sleeping habits (Paakkari et al., 2019).

A suggested model from the School for Health in Europe Network provides an example of the interplay between health literacy, health and education (Okan, Paakkari & Dadaczynski, 2020). It focuses on micro- and meso-level factors but macro-level factors such as national health and education policies, national income, cultural context and institutional set-up are also crucial and should be considered inherent.

6.4.3   *Promoting health and wellbeing at schools*

Education systems and early childhood education and care services are continually searching for ways in which individuals, groups, organizations, communities or institutions can develop the capacities to make decisions and take actions to enjoy good health and wellbeing. New and stronger alliances are needed across sectoral interests to safeguard the creation of more just, inclusive and sustainable societies where everyone can realize their fundamental human rights and unique potential (Kickbusch, 2012).

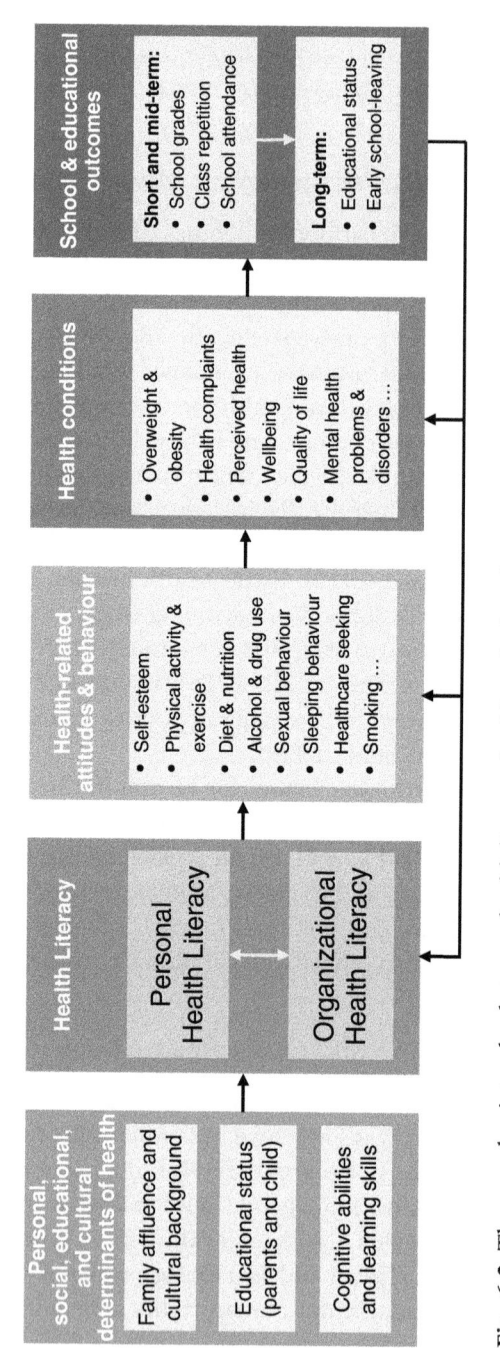

Fig. 6.2 The complex interplay between health literacy, health and education

Source: Okan, Paakkari & Dadaczynski, 2020

Although the relationship between healthy children and able learners has been well established, in practice many children remain insufficiently supported. According to the Child Health Taskforce (2021), estimates in low- and lower middle-income countries have found that annual public spending for health for ages 5–20 is less than US$3 billion. In comparison, public expenditure for education is estimated to be more than US$200 billion. Recognizing that health is a prerequisite for learning, these profound educational investments are likely to fail as inadequate health of children serves as a barrier to learning and development.

Globally, the number of children reaching school age is estimated to be 1.2 billion children, totalling 18% of the world's population, and 88% of these children live in less developed countries where there is a high prevalence of disease and illness. For instance, certain conditions that are prevalent among school-age children and adolescents can impair cognition, attention span and learning. To take one example, the average IQ loss for children with untreated worm infections is estimated to be 3.75 IQ points per child, and the average IQ points lost due to anaemia is even higher.

School Health and Nutrition (SHN) programmes are amongst the most cost-effective interventions that exist to improve both children's education and health. They can add 4 to 6 points to IQ levels, 10% to school participation, and an additional one to two years of education (World Bank, 2011). The focus has shifted significantly in the past two decades from a primarily medical approach to one that is embracing prevention and health promotion, especially among the most disadvantaged and vulnerable groups. School health programmes can cover, for example, both the prevention and treatment of disease and malnutrition in a school setting (Snilstveit et al., 2016). The programmes are designed to promote students' physical, cognitive and social development. They build on existing health infrastructure and community partnerships, as well as a skilled workforce in schools. A pervasive school system provides a platform for delivering simple health interventions to schoolchildren.

By magnitude, since there are more teachers than nurses and more schools than clinics, in cost-benefit analyses school health programmes often compare well with many other education interventions and have the additional advantage of optimizing the benefits of the education already being offered to poor children (Snilstveit et al., 2016). From the health system's point of view, schools represent a cost-effective platform for reaching school-aged children with the interventions they need to achieve their potential human capital. From the educational system's point of view, the delivery of health services ensures that poor health of a child does not become a hindrance to learning, growth and cognitive formation. In this way, investments in school health and nutrition are synergistic and essential to other educational investments focusing on quality and access. Moreover, school health sets the stage for children to thrive and become change agents in their communities.

No education system is effective unless it promotes the health and wellbeing of its students, staff and community. These strong links have never been more visible and compelling than in the context of the COVID-19 pandemic. A multisectoral approach is needed to create optimal learning environments involving active engagement of several ministries, governmental and non-governmental stakeholders, pupils, students and staff as well as the wider school community. The wide-spread movements of Health Promoting Schools and Universities are examples of how the multisectoral approach can be applied in practice. The Health Promoting Schools approach was first articulated by WHO, UNESCO and UNICEF in 1995 and adopted in over 90 countries and territories. However, few countries have implemented it at scale, and even fewer have effectively adapted their education systems to include health promotion. In 2021, a new set of global standards was launched to help countries integrating health promotion into all schools to boost the health and wellbeing of their children (WHO & UNESCO, 2021). The standards highlight these eight action areas:

1. government policies and resources: the whole of government is committed to and invests in making every school a health-promoting school;
2. school policies and resources: the school is committed to and invests in a whole-school approach to being a health-promoting school;
3. school governance and leadership: a whole-school model of school governance and leadership supports a health-promoting school;
4. school and community partnerships: the school is engaged and collaborates with the local community for health-promoting school;
5. school curriculum: the school curriculum supports physical, social-emotional and psychological aspects of student health and wellbeing;

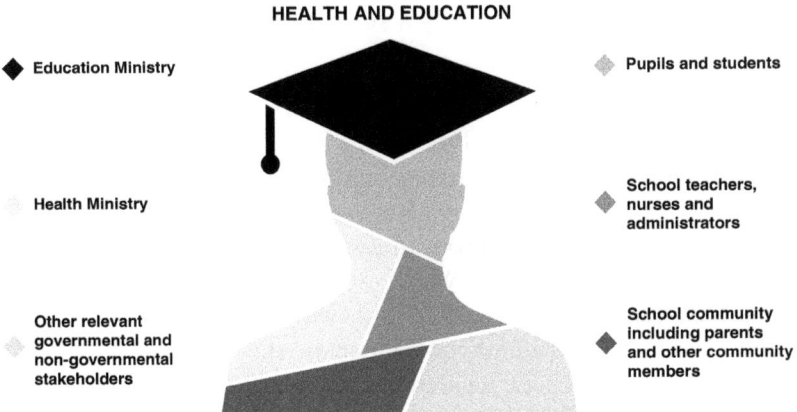

HEALTH AND EDUCATION

◆ Education Ministry

Health Ministry

Other relevant
governmental and
non-governmental
stakeholders

Pupils and students

School teachers,
nurses and
administrators

School community
including parents
and other community
members

Fig. 6.3 Examples of stakeholders safeguarding health in school settings

6. school social-emotional environment: the school has a safe, supportive social-emotional environment;
7. school physical environment: the school has a healthy, safe, secure, inclusive physical environment; and
8. school health services: all students have access to comprehensive school-based or school-linked health services that meet their physical, emotional, psychosocial and educational health care needs.

6.5   Improving the capacity of people in vulnerable situations through health literacy

For certain risk groups, more targeted interventions may be needed. The MILSA initiative is a Swedish example which uses health literacy as a lever for better education and sustainable development among newly arrived refugees and migrants. The MILSA platform is a national educational platform facilitating training on civic literacy and health literacy. It involves courses and engagement of local health mediators that can respond adequately to the needs and concerns of newly arrived refugees to build capacity and help them settle in their new settings. It involves different actors such as municipalities, government institutions and civil society, and focuses on health, human rights and fundamental democratic values, individual rights and responsibilities, the organization of Swedish society and the health system, as well as everyday life in a Swedish context (MILSA, 2018).

6.6   The health workforce as a source of educational capacity

The health workforce serves as a major contribution to achieve the Sustainable Development Goals. Global health mandates and resolutions have consistently emphasized the need for health workforce strengthening through lifelong learning opportunities (WHO, 2020). However, the density of skilled health workers varies greatly, from 106.4 per 10 000 population in the European Region to 14.1 per 10 000 population in the African Region (WHO, 2017). In this regard, scaling up and integrating digital tools for health workforce development have been recommended as a pathway to increase the educational capacity.

A framework has been suggested by WHO (2020) which addresses the external, system-level, institutional and individual factors required to embed information and communication technologies as foundations for maximizing the potential of digital education and reducing the digital divide:

External factors include the level of digital and health literacy of the population, and the extent to which the target population is receptive to adopting innovations and ICT systems, as well as the degree of commitment and support of governmental and nongovernmental actors. The culture and receptiveness of learning audiences to digital education is important to consider; this pertains to the trust that learners implicitly have (or lack) in digital education methods compared with other means available.

System-level factors include the incorporation of health workforce development objectives in long-term plans and evidence-based policy, sufficiency of technical infrastructure, appropriate levels of funding, and robustness of multisectoral collaboration among stakeholders (for example, ministries of health, education, health academic centres, health care delivery organizations, IT companies). Digital education can address the standardization of the quality of curricula and accreditation mechanisms to allow for a uniform assessment of different educational institutions. Similarly, standardizing user interfaces/formats could play an important part in user acceptance.

Institutional factors include the level of organizational ownership, availability of infrastructure, governance, financing and management support, expertise in development of health education curricula and teaching resources using digital tools, and deployment of education modules using appropriate digital health technologies, as well as training plans for developing human resources, teachers and administrators.

Individual factors include the beliefs, attitudes and behaviours of administrators, teachers, students and support staff involved in the educational and technical processes.

A professional, qualified and multidisciplinary workforce, in sufficient numbers, is vital to the organization and management of effective public health systems as a means to respond to the growing threats to population health, to address health inequalities between and within countries, and to develop and implement scientifically based interventions in a timely and appropriate manner within the limits of available resources. Capacity development is the process through which individuals, organizations and societies obtain, strengthen and maintain their capabilities to set and achieve their own development objectives over time. Capacity development goes well beyond the technical cooperation and training approaches that have been associated with "capacity building" in the past. The current health sector has widened their focus to include strengthening of individuals, organizations and the wider environment (or society), and not solely focusing on individuals as in the past.

Constant societal change implies an increased need to update educational sources. For instance, amid the COVID-19 pandemic situation, countries across the world introduced capacity development measures to prevent its spread, increase surveillance capacity, improve contact tracing, and increase isolation and quarantine capacity, as well as augmenting the capacity of hospitals (particularly intensive care units) and staff to effectively manage positive cases. Enhancing health system capacity for the design and implementation of strategies that minimize the impact posed by such crises will remain a critical determinant of progress towards achieving the sustainable development goals (Gera, 2020).

Relying heavily on inter-professional collaborations, there is also growing evidence from developed and developing countries that community-based approaches are effective in improving the public's health for better education. Preventing disease and promoting health calls for a holistic approach to health interventions, including addressing the social determinants of health in which the health force plays a crucial role (Institute of Medicine, 2015).

6.7 The way forward to achieve more co-benefits of health and education for all

Despite shortcomings, the social and economic opportunities derived from the past decades of societal transformation have spurred a growing focus on health and wellbeing in countries around the world. The co-benefits include healthier populations, more efficient public health systems, and decreased literacy and poverty. Taking these benefits into account when planning political priorities and strategies may enable decisionmakers to address multiple social, environmental and economic barriers for better health to achieve better educational outcomes.

The aspects of mental, physical and emotional health are all critical to excellent academic performance. With the development of conducive environments and the nurture of good habits early on in life, there is an increased opportunity to implement an improvement in healthier lifestyles with the added benefit of a progression in educational performance. Countries like Finland and Iceland are frontrunners as they have included health education as part of their primary and secondary school curricula to maximize the co-benefits.

Moreover, the digital revolution has changed the demands for health and education in a contemporary context. Digital literacy is an area that is closely associated with health literacy and the improvement of education across generations. Education is no longer about maths, reading and writing alone; it is about knowing how to learn, de-learn and re-learn new issues relevant for modern living. Applied to health, the COVID-19 pandemic is an example of this perspective. When it appeared as a new condition, societies around the world had to understand its implications and apply new ways of living, such as the use of online services, to curb its impact for maintaining sustainable development.

While most attention has been given to the impact of education on health, advancing health and wellbeing remains a critical pathway to achieve education and lifelong learning. Sustainable development goes hand in hand with increased investments in health literacy, learning for wellbeing and capacity development. To compound the vested interest and impact, it is, therefore, recommended to provide a reorientation of systemic thinking and practice which build on health and wellbeing as central elements of achieving quality education during the life course.

References

Arpino B, Gumà J, Julià A (2018). Early-life conditions and health at older ages: the mediating role of educational attainment, family and employment trajectories. PLoS One, 13(4):e0195320. (https://doi.org/10.1371/journal .pone.0195320)

Child Health Taskforce (2021). School health and nutrition. (https://www .childhealthtaskforce.org/hubs/school-health-and-nutrition)

CSDH (2008). Closing the gap in a generation: health equity through action on the social determinants of health. Final Report of the Commission on Social Determinants of Health. Geneva, World Health Organization.

Dadaczynski K (2012). State of science on the relationship between health and education: An empirical overview and implications for school health promotion [In German]. Gesundheitspsychol, 20:141–53. (https://doi .org/10.1026/0943-8149/a000072)

Dadaczynski K, Rathmann K, Schricker J et al. (2020). Digital health literacy of adolescents. A multi-perspective view from the perspective of students, teachers and school administrators of secondary schools in Hesse [In German]. Fulda.

Fleary SA, Joseph P, Pappagianopoulos JE (2018). Adolescent health literacy and health behaviors: A systematic review. J Adolesc, 62:116–27. (https:// doi.org/10.1016/j.adolescence.2017.11.010)

Gera A (2020). Capacity development of the public health workforce in the current COVID19 era. J Health Commun, 5(6).

Gumà J, Solé-Auró A, Arpino B (2019) . Examining social determinants of health: the role of education, household arrangements and country groups by gender. BMC Public Health, 19:699.

Institute of Medicine (2015). Building Health Workforce Capacity Through Community-Based Health Professional Education: Workshop Summary. Washington, DC: National Academies Press. (https://doi .org/10.17226/18973)

Kickbusch ILSF, Gordon J, O'Toole L (2012). Learning for Wellbeing – a policy priority for children and youth in Europe. A process for change, with the collaboration of Jean Gordon and Linda O'Toole. Drafted on behalf of the Learning for Well-being Consortium of Foundations in Europe, Universal Education Foundation, Meerbeke.

McDaid D (2016). Investing in health literacy: What do we know about the co-benefits to the education sector of actions targeted at children and young people? Copenhagen: European Observatory on Health Systems and Policies.

MILSA (2018). National education platform for civic and health communication [website]. Malmö: County Administrative Board of Skåne. (https://www .lansstyrelsen.se/skane/tjanster/publikationer/milsa–national-education-platform-for-civic-and-health-communication.html, 9 March 2022)

M-POHL (2021). The HLS19 Consortium of the WHO Action Network M-POHL (2021): International Report on the Methodology, Results, and Recommendations of the European Health Literacy Population Survey 2019–2021 (HLS19) of M-POHL. Vienna: Austrian National Public Health Institute.

Okan O, Paakkari L, Dadaczynski K (2020). Health literacy in schools. State of the art. SHE factsheet no. 6. Schools for Health in Europe. (https:// www.schoolsforhealth.org/sites/default/files/editor/fact-sheets/factsheet-2020-english.pdf)

Paakkari LT, Torppa MP, Paakkari O-P et al. (2019). Does health literacy explain the link between structural stratifiers and adolescent health? Eur J Public Health, 29:919–924. (https://doi.org/10.1093/eurpub/ckz011)

Paakkari L, Torppa M, Mazur J et al. (2020). A Comparative Study on Adolescents' Health Literacy in Europe: Findings from the HBSC Study. Int J Environ Res Public Health, 17(10):3543. (https://doi.org/10.3390/ijerph17103543)

Quaglio G et al. (2017). Accelerating the health literacy agenda in Europe. Health promot int, 32(6):1074–1080.

Ross C, Wu C (1995). The links between education and health. Am Sociol Rev, 60(5):719–745. (https://doi.org/10.2307/2096319).

Ross CE, Mirowsky J (2010). Gender and the health benefits of education. Sociol Q, 51:1–19. (https://doi.org/10.1111/j.1533-8525.2009.01164.x).

Ross CE, Masters RK, Hummer RA (2012). Education and the gender gaps in health and mortality. Demography, 49:1157–1183. (https://doi .org/10.1007/s13524-012-0130-z)

Rowlands G, Russell S, O'Donnell A et al. (2018). What is the evidence on existing policies and linked activities and their effectiveness for improving health literacy at national, regional and organizational levels in the WHO European Region? Copenhagen: WHO Regional Office for Europe (Health Evidence Network (HEN) synthesis report 57).

Shih S-F, Liu C-H, Liao L-L et al. (2016). Health literacy and the determinants of obesity. A population based survey of sixth grade school children in Taiwan. BMC Public Health, 16:280. (https://doi.org/10.1186/s12889-016-2879-2)

Snilstveit B et al. (2016). The impact of education programmes on learning and school participation in low-and middle-income countries.

Sørensen K, Okan O (2020). Health Literacy. Health Literacy of children and adolescents in school settings. Global Health Literacy Acad./Fac. of Educational Science, Univ. Bielefeld/Internat. School Health Network.

Sørensen K et al. (2015). Health literacy in Europe: comparative results of the European health literacy survey (HLS-EU). Eur j public health, 25(6):1053–1058.

UNESCO (2017). Education for sustainable development.

UNESCO (2021). Leading SDG 4 – Education 2030. (https://en.unesco.org/themes/education2030-sdg4, 23 August 2021)

United Nations (2015). Transforming our world: the 2030 Agenda for Sustainable Development. Resolution A/70/L.1.

WHO (2017). Framing the health workforce agenda for the Sustainable Development Goals: biennium report 2016–2017 – WHO Health Workforce. Geneva: World Health Organization (WHO/HIS/HWF/biennium report/2017.1). Licence: CC BY-NC-SA 3.0 IGO.

WHO (2019). EUR/RC69/R9 Resolution towards the implementation of health literacy initiatives through the life course. (https://www.euro.who.int/__data/assets/pdf_file/0005/413861/69rs09e_ResolutionHealthLiteracy_190598.pdf)

WHO (2020). Digital education for building health workforce capacity. Geneva: World Health Organization; 2020. Licence: CC BY-NC-SA 3.0 IGO.

WHO (2021). E4As guide for advancing health and sustainable development. Resources and tools for policy development and implementation. Copenhagen: WHO Regional Office for Europe.

WHO Europe (2013). Health literacy: the solid facts.

WHO/UNESCO (2021). Making every school a health-promoting school: global standards and indicators for health-promoting schools and systems. Geneva: World Health Organization and the United Nations Educational, Scientific and Cultural Organization.

World Bank (2011). Rethinking school health: a key component of education for all. New York. (https://schoolsandhealth.net/Shared%20Documents/Downloads/Rethinking%20School%20Health%20A%20key%20component%20of%20Education%20for%20All.pdf)

Zajacova A, Lawrence EM (2018). The relationship between education and health: reducing disparities through a contextual approach. Annu Rev Public Health, 39:273–289. (https://doi.org/10.1146/annurev-publhealth-031816-044628)

7 | *SDG5, gender equality: co-benefits and challenges*

ELLEN KUHLMANN, GABRIELA LOTTA

7.1 Introduction

Universal healthcare coverage (UHC), "Health for all" and "Leaving no one behind" (WHO, 2021) need to include equity of and access for women, men and all other genders. The reverse is true as well: gender equality and human rights need health equity. Assessing policy co-benefits and improving intersectoral governance may help us achieve progress in these areas. This chapter explores the linkages between SDG3 Health and SDG5 "Achieve gender equality and empower all women and girls". We introduce selected sub-goals/targets of the two SDGs and briefly clarify the terms and concepts of gender equality. We argue that health equity and gender equality are "'twin forces" that are historically connected and cannot be separated, creating either strong co-benefits or a "double jeopardy" scenario for health and gender equality. Thus, developments at the crossroads of SDG3 and SDG5 are never "gender neutral" and need attention for two reasons: to strengthen the health policy co-benefits and to prevent and mitigate adverse effects if gender equality is ignored.

The chapter describes the pathways between health and gender equality, taking into account theoretical issues, governance and policy challenges. We introduce a conceptual model of researching co-benefits that expands the focus on macro-level co-benefits towards more complex governance processes and outcomes. Selected empirical case studies consider four major targets of SDG5 and related SDG3 sub-goals, illustrating different scenarios of implementation of health and gender co-benefits in a range of policy and governance contexts.

Our first case study highlights an optimum scenario of co-benefits driven by health policy action, using two mini-case studies as empirical examples: domestic violence against women (Amin, Kismödi & García-Moreno, 2015; WHO, 2002) and training midwives to improve access of migrant women to healthcare (Fair et al., 2021). Both examples are characterized through a global/European approach and a scenario of "high importance" and "low conflict" of SDG3 and SDG5 that supports intersectoral governance. Case study 2 sets the focus on the developments in the health workforce during the coronavirus (COVID-19) pandemic in Brazil (until December 2022, under the Presidency of Bolsonaro), one of the worst hit countries and regions in the world (Lancet, 2021). It illustrates a problematic scenario of political elites strongly contradicting epidemiological facts and public health relevance and ignoring both the population's health and gender equality. The Brazilian case study reflects a "low importance/high (public health) conflict" scenario on the side of the political actors and reveals the "double jeopardy" for gender equality and public health when health policy action co-benefits are lacking. Our final case focuses on the European Union (EU) and a more mixed scenario of "importance" and "conflict" where the results depend on the stakeholder groups. This case sheds light on academia and the science system, where evidence and "epidemiological facts" are produced and leadership is defined. This makes academia an important arena and a major switchboard of SDG co-benefits, including both the substance (research) and the institutions. The example of coronary heart disease reveals the capacity of co-benefits when health action is supported by intersectoral governance and the threats to health and equality if gender is ignored.

The selection of cases seeks to highlight how gender matters in different contexts and how systematic interlinks between the different SDGs may create co-benefits for health care and gender equality. The three scenarios and empirical cases illustrate that governance actions and intersectoral structures (institutional pathways) shape the "windows of opportunity" for co-benefits. Co-benefits remain fragile and contested and need thus to be re-assured, a lesson most recently learned from the COVID-19 pandemic (Kuhlmann et al., 2023; Lotta et al., 2021; Tomsick, Smith & Wenham, 2022; Wenham et al., 2020).

7.2   Background

Strong connections between SDG3 and SDG5 have created intersecting health and gender equality targets (United Nations, 1999). The targets are specified in the SDG sub-goals. We have selected four targets of SDG5 to explore major synergies and interlinks:

- SDG5.1: "End all forms of discrimination against all women and girls everywhere";

- SDG5.2: "Eliminate all forms of violence against all women and girls in the public and private spheres";
- SDG5.5: "Ensure women's full and effective participation and equal opportunities for leadership at all levels of decision-making in political, economic and public life"; and
- SDG5.6: "Ensure universal access to sexual and reproductive health and reproductive rights" (https://www.undp.org/sustainable-development-goals#gender-equality).

Some SDG3 targets are explicitly linked to gender equality (Gupta et al., 2019). These include SDG3.1 "Reduce maternal mortality", SDG3.7 "Universal access to sexual and reproductive health care services" (WHO Europe, 2017) and SDG3C "Support to health workforce" (WHO Europe, 2018). More recently, Target 16.1 "Reduce violence everywhere" has been added, arguing among others that "[G]endered social and cultural norms and concepts of masculinity increase the risk of violence" (WHO, 2020a). SDG3.8 "Achieve universal health coverage" highlights the need to "leave no one behind" and pays greater attention to the needs of vulnerable groups; this also provides a platform for including gender equality more explicitly and addressing intersecting social inequalities.

Some international declarations and commissions on gender equality are explicitly linked to health and the SDGs (Gupta et al., 2019; United Nations, 1999). The *Gender Equality, Norms and Health Steering Committee* provides a good example of how intersectoral governance may create co-benefits driven by health action. The Committee highlights that "[R]esearch, health systems, policies, and programmes can reduce gender inequalities, shift gender norms, and improve health" (Gupta et al., 2019). Similarly, the *Women and Gender Equity Knowledge Network of the WHO Commission on Social Determinants of Health* has previously argued that "taking action to improve gender equity in health and to address women's health is one of the most direct and potent ways to reduce health inequities and ensure effective use of health resources" (Sen, Östlin & George, 2007). The *Spotlight Initiative* joined forces with the United Nations and the European Commission in a global partnership (supported by WHO) to "eliminate all forms of violence against women and girls", demonstrating how action can be taken to improve "Health for All" (Spotlight Initiative, 2021). More generally, the *European Pillar of*

Social Rights Action Plan demonstrates the interlinks between gender, health and other sectors (European Commission, 2021a).

Health sector actions may support gender equality (see, for example, Abdool, García-Moreno & Amin, 2012; Amin, Kismödi & García-Moreno, 2015; Kuhlmann & Annandale, 2015; Morgan et al., 2021; Takemoto et al., 2021) and co-benefits are strongest "when they engage multiple stakeholders from different sectors" (Gupta et al., 2019). However, co-benefits are rarely considered in a more pro-active manner as an important policy concept and they are still poorly researched.

Some brief clarification regarding the terminology may be helpful (Annandale & Kuhlmann, 2012; Kuhlmann, 2009; Wenham, 2021). Historically, the distinction between sex (more related to biological dimensions) and gender (more related to social conditions and identity) has helped to explore how differences between women and men are socially constructed. However, since the 1990s feminists and scholars of postmodern theories have illuminated the connections (for example, Haraway, 1988) and questioned the sex/gender and culture/nature distinctions (Kuhlmann, 2009), also highlighting intersectionality of social inequalities (Lotta et al., 2021). Notwithstanding the important theoretical differences, the categories of sex and gender are increasingly perceived as fluid and interconnected, and this is especially relevant in relation to health. For the purpose of this chapter – and in line with SDG5 – we utilize "gender" as an umbrella term, which includes biological dimensions as well as women, men and other sexes/genders and their sexual orientations (often summarized as LGBTQ – lesbian, gay, bisexual, transsexual, queer – or non-binary people). We also follow the SDG5 targets by focusing on women's/girls' health, while acknowledging that a gender approach and attention to co-benefits are also relevant in the group of men/boys as well as in relation to sexual minority groups (Morgan et al., 2021; Rice et al., 2021).

We refer to a non-binary concept of sex-gender – including women, men and other genders – and to intersectionality as an approach:

"wherein gender intersects with other social markers of power, such as race, age, and income, to create clustered relative advantage or disadvantage that gives rise to power dynamics and hierarchies among boys and men and girls and women, not just between them" (Gupta et al., 2019).

The strong connections between SDG3 and SDG5 have created specific conditions of co-benefits. One key characteristic is the *embodied* nature of the sex–gender–health connections (Kuhlmann, 2009). Another important issue is the *intersectionality* of gender with other forms of social inequality (Gupta et al., 2019; Krieger & Davey Smith, 2004). Intersecting social inequalities may create marginalized groups and may thus have negative effects on the physical and mental health of the people affected, as well as on societal coherence and resilience of health systems and societies. A third characteristic is the *gender–power nexus*, pushing women more often to the bottom and men to the top of societies and marginalizing those who do not fit a binary gender order, such as LGBTQ people (European Network against Racism, 2021; Paine, 2018). In relation to policy and governance, the two SDGs draw on largely similar policy approaches of *mainstreaming* major targets into different policy areas. SDG3 is informed by Health in All Policies (Leppo et al., 2013) and SDG5 by "gender mainstreaming" (Council of Europe, 1998; Kuhlmann & Annandale, 2012). Also, UHC is still an "unfinished journey" (Rajan, Richiardi & McKee, 2020) and much the same applies to gender mainstreaming (Allotey & Denton, 2020). Thus, co-benefits should be considered as a process – bringing the role of actors and stakeholder groups into play – and a policy tool rather than an outcome.

7.3   Pathways between health action and co-benefits

The procedural nature of SDG3 and SDG5 co-benefits, together with the interconnectedness, embodiment and intersectionality of health and sex/gender, makes it difficult to identify linear relationships and causal pathways (Kuhlmann & Annandale, 2015). In some areas, health action and gender equality co-benefits may be amalgamated; this applies, for instance, to maternity care as a typical SDG3 and SDG5 co-benefit. In most other areas, things are more complicated and less positive.

Major challenges to the development of intersectoral governance and the creation of co-benefits are arising from the "embodied" connections between health and sex-gender. These conditions bear the risks of either reinforcing differences as "natural facts" and essentialist attitudes (for example, "hardiness" of men, "caring attitudes" of women) or hiding gendered power relations and inequalities behind seemingly "gender-neutral" approaches. A neutrality paradigm is based on a White, male, heterosexual person, thus creating disadvantages for all women and "double jeopardy" or even "triple jeopardy" for female members of ethnic minority groups and LGBTQ people. Neutrality may also threaten men who do not fit, or do not want to fit into the norms of "hegemonic masculinities" (Connell & Messerschmidt, 2005). Assuming neutrality inevitably excludes many people. It creates health risks, most often for women and girls, but in some areas (such as mental health) also for men (Kuhlmann & Annandale, 2015; Morgan et al., 2021; Ovseiko et al., 2017; Rice et al., 2021).

The "coronavirus politics" (Greer et al., 2021) have added new examples of gender-blindness and policy failures that impact women/girls and minority groups most, but may also create risks for men (European Parliament, 2021; Global Health 50/50, 2021; Morgan et al., 2021; Tomsick, Smith & Wenham, 2022; UNDP-UN Women, 2020). For instance, lockdown policies have increased the risks of sexual and domestic violence (WHO, 2020a), they have disrupted reproductive health care services (Bojovic, Stanisljevic & Giunti, 2021; Takemoto et al., 2021) and disadvantaged female health care workers (HCW) and female-dominated health care sectors in relation to pandemic protection and preparedness (Lotta et al., 2021; Shamseer et al., 2021; WHO, 2020b) (for an overview, see Kuhlmann et al., 2023).

New inequalities often emerged despite strong legal gender equality frameworks and anti-discrimination policies, a situation observed, for example, within the EU (Council of Europe, 1998; European Commission, 2020). For instance, women's jobs are more at risk during the pandemic and for those "who remain in employment, their greater care obligations are forcing them to cut down on paid working hours or to extend total working hours (paid and unpaid) to unsustainable levels" (ILO, 2020). The International Labour Market Organization calls upon policymakers to put "gender equality at the core of the emergency and recovery efforts to avoid long-term damage to women's job prospects and to build back better and fairer" (ILO, 2020; see also Gupta, 2019).

A WHO country briefing provides another illustrative example of how to create co-benefits and implement intersectoral governance in the health care system in times of COVID-19. The WHO advises Member States "to incorporate a focus on gender into their COVID-19 responses in order to ensure that public health policies and measures to curb the epidemic take account of gender and how it interacts with other areas of inequality" (WHO, 2020b). Although the briefing does not use the term, it clearly refers to co-benefits and reveals supportive conditions of intersectoral action.

7.3.1   *Governance and implementation challenges*

An intersectoral governance approach is important, but is no free ticket to co-benefits. Strong power and interest-driven politics and contradictory developments in the health care system and society shape the implementation processes at the crossroads of SDG3 and SDG5, thus challenging governance and policy outcomes. For instance, successful efforts on the macro-level of governance through equal opportunity laws and joint funding sources, for example, observed in the EU (European Commission, 2020), may be hampered by "organizational plaques" of "old-boys-networks" (Sen, Östlin & George, 2007) or by new performance management schemes that benefit men more than women, for example in academic health care settings (Kuhlmann et al., 2017).

Successful macro-level efforts may also be weakened or even blocked on the micro-level through cultural, ethnic or religious stereotypes and attitudes, for example, if women are prevented from developing leadership skills and men from developing caring skills, or if women's sexual and reproductive rights are denied and sexual violence justified as cultural practice (Zuccala & Horton, 2018). Governing the implementation of SDGs in ways that enhance co-benefits, therefore, needs a flexible intersectoral approach and knowledge of processes and actors at macro- and micro-levels and in different policy areas.

7.3.2   *Policy challenges*

The SDGs and mainstreaming policies have spotlighted gender relations and helped bring equity and equality to the policy agenda (Council of Europe, 1998; Kuhlmann & Annandale, 2012; United Nations, 1999). However, no country has achieved the goals (Allotey & Denton, 2020). Major challenges, such as preventing sexual violence, continue to persist (Amin, Kismödi & García-Moreno, 2015; WHO, 2020a) and the COVID-19 pandemic has caused a global backlash in all areas of gender equality (Global Health 50/50, 2021; Lotta et al., 2021; Morgan et al., 2021). Some of these problems are rooted in the SDGs and the gender blindness of health policymaking (Hawkes & Buse,

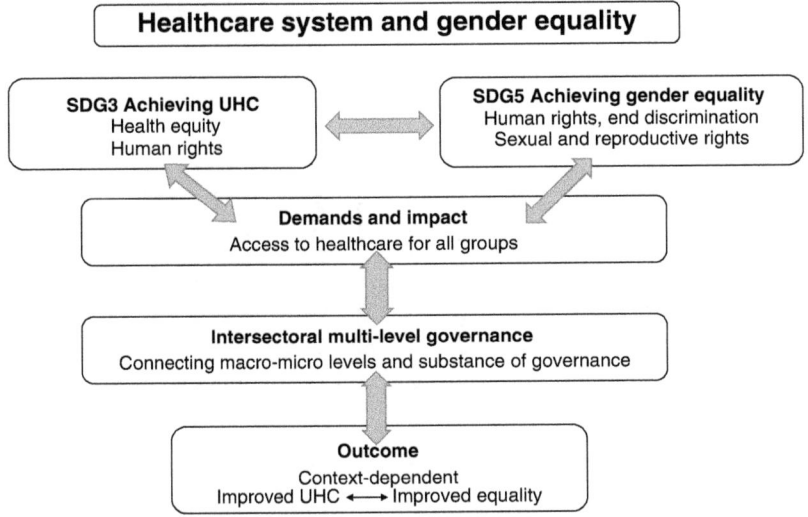

Fig. 7.1 Connected pathways of SDG3 and SDG5 co-benefits

2013; Kuhlmann & Annandale, 2015; Zuccala & Horton, 2018), while others are caused by a lack of attention to conflicting interests and diverse needs. Fig. 7.1 introduces a conceptual framework for assessing health and gender action co-benefits in context.

Intersectoral multi-level governance in health care can be operationalized through a number of tools and every tool can be, and should be, utilized to support the creation of SDG5 and SDG3 co-benefits, as defined by gender mainstreaming (Abdool, García-Moreno & Amin, 2012; Kuhlmann & Annandale, 2012). For instance, the "Strategy for integrating gender analysis and actions into the work of WHO", reproducing resolution WHA 60.25, calls for incorporating gender equality in health policies, programmes, research and planning processes in any area and at all levels. Mainstreaming must consider the entire process of design, implementation, monitoring and evaluation of policies and programmes in all political, economic and social spheres (WHO, 2009).

Table 7.1 below provides an overview of the tools for possible governance actions to support the creation of co-benefits, illustrating that co-benefits are embedded in gender mainstreaming and SDG5. However, the implementation of "possible" governance actions depends on contexts and may be constrained in many ways. As we put it in

Table 7.1 *Possible governance actions to support co-benefits between SDG5 and SDG3*

Tools			Possible governance actions with these tools								
			Goals and targets	Evidence support	Policy guidance	Implementation and management	Coordination	Advocacy	Monitoring and evaluation	Financial support	Legal mandate
	Plan	Plan	X	X	X	X	X	X	X	X	X
	Indicators and targets	Indicators	X	X	X	X	X	X	X	X	X
		Targets	X	X	X	X	X	X	X	X	X
	Budgeting	Pooled budget	X	X	X	X	X	X	X	X	X
		Shared objectives	X	X	X	X	X	X	X	X	X
		Coordinated budgeting	X	X	X	X	X	X	X	X	X
	Organization	Ministerial linkages	X	X	X	X	X	X	X	X	X
		Specific ministers	X	X	X	X	X	X	X	X	X
		Organization	X	X	X	X	X	X	X	X	X
		Legislative committees	X	X	X	X	X	X	X	X	X
		Interdepartmental committees/units	X	X	X	X	X	X	X	X	X
		Departmental mergers	X	X	X	X	X	X	X	X	X
		Civic engagement	X	X	X	X	X	X	X	X	X
	Accountability	Transparent data	X	X	X	X	X	X	X	X	X
		Regular reporting	X	X	X	X	X	X	X	X	X
		Independent agency/evaluators	X	X	X	X	X	X	X	X	X
		Support for civil society	X	X	X	X	X	X	X	X	X
		Legal rights	X	X	X	X	X	X	X	X	X

Source: Authors' elaboration, based on McQueen et al., 2012

our introduction, health equity and gender equality are "'twin forces" creating either strong co-benefits or a "double jeopardy" scenario for health and gender equality.

7.4 Case study 1: health action creating co-benefits to gender equality and women's health

We have selected two mini-case studies to illustrate an optimum scenario of health action creating gender equality co-benefits with a focus on women's health. The examples refer to large multi-country projects that implemented intersectoral governance elements aiming to improve women's health. In addition, evaluations of outcomes and transferability are available, which are lacking in most other cases.

The first case reflects the intersectionality of gender and race/ethnicity and the opportunities of creating co-benefits for socially disadvantaged and marginalized groups of women within the EU. The EU project *Operational Refugee and Migrant Maternal Approach* (Box 7.1) aimed to provide intercultural training for midwives and to establish partnerships between health professionals and service users (Fair et al., 2021; ORAMMA, 2020; Petelos et al., 2019; WHO, 2019). The project responds to the growing demand for better health care services and UHC for pregnant women of minority groups.

Box 7.1 Operational Refugee and Migrant Maternal Approach (ORAMMA)

"The project ... has a vision to develop an operational and strategic approach in order to promote safe motherhood, to improve access and delivery of maternal health care for refugee and migrant women and to improve maternal health equality within the European Union. Moreover, the project will increase awareness, commitment and action towards improving maternal health of refugees in the EU. There is an increasing need for a prompt, coordinated, and effective response for all migrant and refugee pregnant and lactating women with newborn babies. Migrant and refugee women face specific health risks and challenges during perinatal period. ... The ORAMMA project will develop, pilot, implement and evaluate by comparative analysis an integrated and cost-effective approach on safe motherhood provision for migrant and refugee women."

Source: ORAMMA, 2019

This example shows an amalgamation of SDG3 targets captured in sub-goals 3.1 "Reduce maternal mortality" and 3.7 "Universal access to sexual and reproductive health care services"' and SDG5 target "Ensure universal access to sexual and reproductive health and reproductive rights". In addition, it considers inclusiveness and support for minority groups. A recent evaluation highlights that the "training improved midwives' knowledge and self-perceived cultural competence in three European countries with differing contexts and workforce provision", although the actual impact in the provision of care and the long-term effects remain to be seen (Fair et al., 2021; see also Petelos et al., 2019).

The second example takes a global approach and highlights policy pathways and strong co-benefits in the prevention of domestic violence against women. Box 7.2 refers to an international WHO project (Amin, Kismödi & García-Moreno, 2015; WHO, 2002), exploring how health action can enhance change in other areas of gender equality. This project makes the implementation pathways of co-benefits created through health policy action visible (although it does not explicitly refer to a co-benefit approach). It demonstrates the transferability across countries and regions of the world, with a focus on low- and middle-income countries.

Box 7.2 Women's health and domestic violence against women: the WHO multi-country study

"The WHO multi-country study brought together researchers, women's organizations working on violence against women, and policymakers from ten countries to develop policy and action-oriented research to measure the magnitude, risk and protective factors and consequences of violence against women. The study was designed to engage with local women's organizations, build capacity, generate dialogue among the different partners and generate new information that could lead to policy change. The implementation of the study led to an increased awareness about violence against women among researchers as well as among the women interviewed. It led to the inclusion of violence against women in national and educational policy agendas of several Ministries of Health. For example, in Brazil, domestic and sexual violence was incorporated as a new subject in the training programme for family physicians. In Peru violence against women was incorporated into a master's course on reproductive health. And in Thailand the institutions responsible for implementation of the study established networks and

---

Box 7.2 (cont.)

became sources of information on the issue. The results of the study also contributed to dialogue with policymakers and the public and to legal and policy discussions. For example, in Thailand the data contributed to discussions on a domestic violence bill, which, based on the study results, included provisions for marital rape that were not considered earlier. In Namibia, the study contributed to discussions on the anti-rape bill. In Maldives, the results were used to launch a campaign to stop violence against women that included participation of the Prime Minister and other dignitaries. In short, the research itself became an intervention with important benefits for driving policy changes in addition to the production of data."

Source: Amin, Kismödi & García-Moreno, 2015:605–606, with reference to WHO, 2002

These two mini cases reflect a scenario of "high salience" and "low conflict" that supports intersectoral governance action and reinforces co-benefits. In both cases, the governance contexts are similar and characterized through a legal mandate, joint funding, strong advocacy and public engagement, among others (Table 7.1). Both projects apply a participatory governance approach, most strongly emphasized by the WHO project. ORAMMA aims to "establish partnerships" between midwives and the pregnant migrant refugee women, while the WHO project highlights engagement with "local women's organizations", "dialogue among the different partners", also including health professionals, policymakers and the public. Strong stakeholder involvement in all stages of the project appears to be an important factor of successful outcomes (Amin, Kismödi & García-Moreno, 2015). Especially, health professionals can be "change agents" and generally play an important role in policy implementation (Gofen & Lotta, 2021). Thus, the creation of co-benefits reflects key characteristics of "good governance" (Greer et al., 2019).

A number of specific conditions apply, however, which may challenge the co-benefits. In particular, sexual and reproductive rights are highly contested, as the attacks on the rights of LGBQT people in Hungary, or the new restriction of abortion rights in Poland, for instance, demonstrate. Both are EU countries and formally accountable to gender equality law and policy, yet national right-wing and populist politics, together with cultural and religious belief systems, are more powerful than EU laws. The implementation of intersectoral governance may therefore be more challenging and constrained (UNDP-UN Women, 2020) than a supportive policy scenario and close linkages between SDG3 and SDG5 suggest.

Furthermore, the COVID-19 pandemic has taught us that co-benefits are not a stable outcome (WHO, 2020c), but must be continuously confirmed and rearranged. Health care workers, especially women in the health workforce networks, play an important role as gender equality advocates in these processes, as co-benefits are contested and may easily be blocked by public health emergencies perceived to be more relevant than gender equality. This can be observed during the pandemic in different policy contexts and even in countries with institutional paths of intersectoral governance and established mainstreaming policies (Bojovic, Stanisljevic & Giunti, 2021; Takemoto et al., 2021). The major outcomes of these cases include strengthening awareness of the health needs of women and creating pathways towards intersectoral and participatory governance. Such pathways can also contribute more generally towards compliance to public health measures, trust in governments and institutions, and increased preparedness and resilience.

A policy scenario of high salience and low conflict of SDG5 targets increases the likelihood that available tools are used effectively and governance actions support the creation of co-benefits (Table 7.1).

7.5   Case study 2: health care workers during the COVID-19 pandemic in Brazil and gender (in)equality

The Brazilian case about health care workers during the COVID-19 pandemic is a good illustration of a problematic situation, considering the lack of focus on gender inequalities. During the pandemic and the period of the Bolsonara presidency, gender issues were made invisible and the Brazilian health workforce, mostly composed of women, was exposed to risky conditions.

Brazil is a middle-income country, which was until December 2022 governed by a right-wing populist president who denied the threats of the pandemic and refused to take action to protect the population. Consequently, Brazil is one of the countries with the highest incidence and death rates of COVID-19 globally (Lotta & Kuhlmann, 2021; Lotta et al., 2021; Rocha et al., 2021) and was ranked as the worst-case worldwide in facing the pandemic (Lowy Institute, 2021). This was far from expected, as Brazil has one of the world's biggest public health systems and high expertise in dealing with epidemics (WHO, 2020c).

However, the strong populism and lack of public health action have hampered the appropriate protection of health and care workers (HCWs). Four rounds of surveys conducted during 2020 and 2021 show this scenario: in April 2021, around 50% of the HCWs had not yet received personal protective equipment (PPE) during the pandemic; only 27% received training and 15% were tested. Consequently, 70% did not feel prepared to work during the pandemic, 88% feel afraid, and 80% have mental health issues due to the pandemic (Lotta et al., 2021). These numbers remained almost the same during the 14 months of the pandemic, evidencing the lack of government efforts.

These data confirm the widespread disregard for HCWs during the pandemic. However, if we disaggregate the data by gender, we see clear differences. As in other countries, more than 70% of the Brazilian health workforce is composed of women and the effects of the pandemic and the lack of policies surrounding HCWs disproportionately impact women. Data from April 2021 show, for example, that women receive less PPE, less training and fewer tests than men; the differences are even greater when including race issues. Black women are the most affected by the pandemic, while White men have the best conditions among the HCWs. For example, while 43% of White men received training, only 21% of Black women did. One of the consequences of these inequalities is that 58% of the HCWs who died during the pandemic were women (Lotta et al., 2021).

Gender inequalities do not only appear in the field of employment, but also in domestic work. Several researchers indicated that the pandemic overloaded women's work with domestic care. This also happened with HCWs. While 51% of the women said they were working more than 14 hours overtime in domestic work during the pandemic, 39% of men reported the same data.

These findings clearly suggest that the lack of attention towards gender issues surrounding HCWs has a higher and more negative impact on women than on men. However, it is important to place this in a broader discussion of gender issues in the Brazilian government that was in office until December 2022. The Brazilian president Jair Bolsonaro was misogynistic, as evidenced in several sexist and homophobic speeches that he was not ashamed to declare. Recently, an analysis of federal policies revealed an explicit misogynistic commonality (Ventura et al., 2021). For example, in April 2021, the health ministry started telling women not to get pregnant during the pandemic, considering the high death rates in Brazil – 80% of all pregnant women killed by COVID-19 worldwide were Brazilian. However, the government did not provide any tools for them to postpone pregnancy (Ventura et al., 2021) and primary health care policies were dismantled (Lotta et al., 2021; see also Kuhlmann et al., 2023). These data show how gender inequalities experienced by HCWs are not exclusive to this professional category. Gender inequalities were structural in this government.

Populism generally opposes gender equality and often attacks minority rights. Within a climate of political attacks and structural ignorance, gender and social inequalities were largely invisible. The Brazilian case evidences this process. This has caused a lack of protection, especially for women and minority groups, and reinforced vulnerabilities in the health workforce. Taking the appropriate action in the health sector would have greatly helped reduce the health risks for female HCWs and those belonging to minority groups, yet the government failed to do so.

The Brazilian case illustrates a scenario of low political salience and subsequently low conflict due to a lack of attention and visibility of inequalities. It also reveals that "salience" is value-based and highly context-dependent. Low political salience and low conflict, as perceived by the elites, strongly contradicts epidemiological conditions and health and societal salience. Consequently, conflict of interests and countervailing powers are embedded in this scenario and might enhance resistance. A climate of populist political attacks combined with an authoritarian government generally hampers intersectoral governance. If action is lacking in both health and gender equality, there is no opportunity for creating co-benefits and using the tools shown in Table 7.1.

However, the strong public health expertise of the Brazilian health care system has established pathways to implement co-benefits, which may be activated to some degree. Especially relevant are established systems of public statistics/research, monitoring and evaluation, as the empirical data confirm. These systems must also improve transparency in sharing data and global health implications, as well as infrastructures to generate them. There are also some formal connections between ministries (even if currently silenced) and most importantly, strong public and stakeholder engagement action might be mobilized if the conflicts increase (Lotta et al., 2022). These conditions might provide hypothetical pathways of co-benefits. However, currently the major outcome is a reinforcement of gender inequality through structural ignorance of population health and gender equality. This has left the HCWs without adequate protection, threatening women, most strongly migrant female HCWs, more than the male groups, the "double" and "triple" jeopardy.

7.6 Case study 3: gender equality in the health science system

The science system is a switchboard of health and gender equality. Medicine, in particular, is furnished with public trust and power to define sex, gender and health and its relationships. The science system produces both the elites that populate politics and the evidence to inform policymakers and practitioners. However, science has been deaf to the calls for gender equality and diversity (Ovseiko et al., 2016). The foundation of modern medicine tells a story of exclusion and "othering" of women, sexual minorities and non-White people, and public health and epidemiology have sadly contributed to the legitimization of inequalities (Krieger & Davey Smith, 2004; Kuhlmann, 2009). We consider global developments but explore the pathways with a focus on the EU and its equal opportunity policies. Key legal elements include, for instance, sexual and reproductive health and rights (SDG5.6; for details, see EUPHA Statement on sexual and reproductive health and rights, 2021) and "effective participation and equal opportunities for leadership at all levels of decision-making in political, economic and public life" (SDG5.5).

Historically the "neutrality" paradigm of science created an invincible bastion, protecting White male elites and the global North against "unpleasant truths" of gender and race assessments and the needs of the global South (Hawkes & Buse, 2013; see also Haraway, 1988). The situation changed when women entered health professions in larger numbers and increased the power of their voice in health research, both as researchers and as users. Here, research into coronary heart disease was one of the milestones, opening new opportunities for gender-sensitive health care and for an emergent field of "gender medicine" (Wenger, 2012). Since the 1990s, large clinical trials show that seemingly gender-neutral diagnosis and treatment of coronary heart disease focus on men and threaten the health of women (for an overview, see for example, GENCAD, 2017; Hulley et al., 1998; Wenger, 2012).

> "In 2003, the Agency for Healthcare Research and Quality Report on the Diagnosis and Treatment of CHD in women, a systematic review of relevant research, concluded that most contemporary recommendations for prevention, diagnostic testing, and medical and surgical treatments of CHD in women were extrapolated from studies conducted predominantly in middle-aged men, with resultant fundamental knowledge gaps regarding the biology, clinical manifestations, and optimal management strategies for women ... Despite their burden of CVD, women remain underrepresented in clinical trials (27% of patients in mixed-sex 1997–2006 National Institutes of Health trials); even when included, women are disadvantaged by absence of sex-specific analyses." (Wenger, 2012).

More recently, attention to the intersections of gender and the non-White and minority groups has increased. For instance, an Australian study revealed that,

> "[I]ndigenous status was associated with more than twice the risk of long-term mortality during a median of 5 years of follow-up, independent of age, comorbidities, presentation, socioeconomic status, and geographical remoteness ... Indigenous patients were younger, more often women." (Dawson, Burchill & O'Brien, 2021).

Like case study 2, this research, too, reveals a "triple jeopardy" of gender and race/ethnicity.

Lessons learned from coronary heart disease research enhanced, for the first time, a chance in clinical guidelines to respond more adequately to women's health needs (GENCAD, 2017). The global nature of medicine helped accelerate and spread gender-sensitive research evidence around the globe, even in countries that lack equal opportunity rights. Next to global transferability, the co-benefits of health action in the field of coronary heart disease spilled over to other areas of health care and policy and even beyond, including those concerned with men's health (Ovseiko et al., 2016). For instance, sex-disaggregated data are now collected and strengthened in many areas of health care (for example, the OECD has significantly increased its data sources), many disciplines have introduced gender-sensitive clinical guidelines and some are monitoring and evaluating the implementation. So, health action co-benefits enhanced transformations towards gender equality, although gender and diversity are still not adequately and effectively addressed (Bambra, Albani & Franklin, 2021; Kuhlmann & Annandale, 2015; Morgan et al., 2021) and a gender leadership gap in academic medicine persists (Kuhlmann et al., 2017).

This case study reflects a scenario of middle-to-strong political salience supported by global research and policy frameworks and by legal action in the EU, in particular, equal opportunity laws implemented through the EU Treaties (Council of Europe, 1998; European Commission, 2020) and translated into Member States' law (albeit in different ways). Intersectoral governance pathways were created on different levels and by a range of diverse stakeholders including public, private and advocacy groups (Table 7.1). Key issues include, for instance, the establishment of "gender mainstreaming" as a global strategy (Allotey & Denton, 2020; United Nations, 1999), the implementation of specific EU and national research programmes and new funding models of "gender budgeting" which connected gender equality goals to financial incentives and shared budgets. Participatory governance and stakeholder engagement were strong elements in some areas (such as maternity care), but poorly developed in most areas of science (Ovseiko et al., 2016).

Macro-level and transnational support structures are helpful, but conflicts may persist at meso- and micro-levels of the health care and science systems as well as in the attitudes of people, outflanking equal opportunity laws and hampering co-benefits. This situation can currently be observed in Europe (and in other countries), where the COVID-19 pandemic has heightened the pressures on the health systems and caused a strong backlash in health equity and gender equality (European Parliament, 2021), also exacerbating intersecting social inequalities (Kuhlmann et al., 2023).

Lack of attention to gender equality in health action has an impact on various levels. It hampers the "production" of knowledge: for example, vaccines are not sufficiently tested for pregnant women. Vijayasingham and colleagues (2021) further highlight that:

"of nearly 2500 COVID-19-related studies, less than 5% of investigators had pre-planned for sex-disaggregated data analysis in their studies, although there are important hints that women and men respond differently to vaccines: Previous influenza vaccine research suggests that women can produce the same immunological response to half-dose vaccine as men do to full dose." (Vijayasingham et al., 2021)

Missing gender sensitivity also affects the "'knowledge producers" themselves, the health professionals: the pandemic threatens the entire health workforce but female HCWs most strongly, as mentioned previously (Shamseer et al., 2021; see also, ILO, 2020) and addressed in more detail by the Brazilian case study.

In case study 3, major outcomes are legally defined gender equality frameworks and changing knowledge systems that support health action co-benefits, such as the implementation of gender-sensitive clinical guidelines. However, elites still dominate knowledge production, while women and minority groups are less well represented, thus facing higher conflicts especially during major public health emergencies like the COVID-19 pandemic.

The examples highlight that governance actions for gender equality must consider both institutions/structures and processes, including the production of data and scientific evidence. This makes the possibilities for creating co-benefits highly context-dependent, shaped to a large degree by stakeholder interests and established coordination across sectors and levels. Governance actions may integrate a wide range of available tools (Table 7.1), but they may also be constrained by policy contexts that ignore the goals of SDG5. The latter scenario is currently demonstrated by the COVID-19 pandemic policies.

7.7   Conclusions

The range of different scenarios (Table 7.2) displayed within this chapter highlight the importance of policy contexts. Our collection of cases provides further information as to *how* context shapes intersectoral governance and the implementation processes of co-benefits. Health policy interventions may create co-benefits especially if flanked by comprehensive intersectoral governance and institutional paths that connect action not only between sectors, but also across the levels and the substance of governance (for example, law and policy, health professional groups, micro-level cultural attitudes) (Fig. 7.1). Strong and diverse stakeholder involvement on all levels of governance appears to be a key condition for achieving positive outcomes. Scenarios 1 and 3

Table 7.2 *The context of policy and implementation of health and gender co-benefits*

EU, migrant maternity care		Conflict	
		Low	High
Political importance	High	X	
	Low		

Brazil, health care workers		Conflict	
		Low	High
Political importance	High		(public health) X
	Low	(politics) X	

EU, gender and science		Conflict	
		Low	High
Political importance	High	X (those in power)	X (women, minority groups)
	Low		

Source: authors' own table, adapted from Page (2005).

explore the pathways between health and gender equality co-benefits mainly through positive examples (benefits) and scenario 2 does so through negative examples (jeopardy). However, all scenarios reveal that established pathways may collapse under pressure, making co-benefits a volatile outcome and a contested policy terrain, as demonstrated most recently by the COVID-19 pandemic (Kuhlmann et al., 2023; Lotta et al., 2021).

The COVID-19 pandemic and the "coronavirus politics" (Greer et al., 2021) have added a new chapter to the health and gender co-benefits. The *Pan-European Commission on Health and Sustainable Development* (2021) is just one of many examples demonstrating how gender equality was "'forgotten" during a major public health crisis (for example, see, for the WHO, Tomsick, Smith & Wenham, 2022). A backlash in gender equality during the COVID-19 pandemic is increasingly documented (Kuhlmann et al., 2023; Lotta et al., 2021; Wenham et al., 2020). As a report by the European Commission shows, the pandemic was "markedly slowing the reported average progress" and 2020 data showed "a clear deterioration for individual indicators" (European Commission, 2021b).

Bringing a gender lens to the debate over SDG co-benefits raises more general questions about universalist policy concepts, which assume "neutrality" and do not adequately respond to policy contexts and the diverse needs and interests of the actors. There is a need for fresh approaches to the SDGs that pay more attention to gender equality and intersectionality, and that better capture and address the importance of participatory governance. The "unfinished journey to universal health care" (Rajan, Richiardi & McKee, 2020) would greatly benefit from a gender-sensitive lens and mainstreaming approach, while co-benefits provide an important policy tool to speed up this journey.

Acknowledgement

We wish to thank Elena Petelos and the editors for their very helpful suggestions.

References

Abdool SN, García-Moreno C, Amin A (2012). Gender equity and international health policy planning. In: Kuhlmann E, Annandale E (eds) The Palgrave Handbook of Gender and Healthcare, second edition. Basingstoke: Palgrave; 36–55.

Allotey P, Denton F (2020). Challenges and priorities for delivering on the Beijing Declaration and Platform for Action 25 years on. Lancet, 396:1053–1054.

Amin A, Kismödi E, García-Moreno C (2015). Addressing violence against women in health policies. In: Kuhlmann E, Blank RH, Bourgeault I et al. (eds) The Palgrave International Handbook of Healthcare Policy and Governance. Basingstoke: Palgrave; 597–614.

Annandale E, Kuhlmann E (2012). Gender and healthcare: the future. In: Kuhlmann E, Annandale E (eds) The Palgrave Handbook of Gender and Healthcare, second edition. Basingstoke: Palgrave; 505–520.

Bambra C, Albani V, Franklin P (2021). The COVID-19 gender health paradox. Scand J Public Health, 49:17–26.

Bojovic N, Stanisljevic J, Giunti G (2021). The impact of COVID-19 on abortion access: insights from the European Union and the United Kingdom. Health Policy, 125:841–858.

Connell RW, Messerschmidt JW (2005). Hegemonic masculinities: rethinking the concept. Gend Soc, 19(6):829–859.

Council of Europe (1998). Gender Mainstreaming. Conceptual Framework, Methodology and Presentation of Good Practice, Final Report (EG-S-MS). Strasbourg: Council of Europe.

Dawson LP, Burchill L, O'Brien J (2021). Differences in outcome of percutaneous coronary intervention between Indigenous and non-Indigenous people in Victoria, Australia: a multicentre, prospective, observational, cohort study. Lancet Global Health, 9(9):e1296–e1304. (https://doi.org/10.1016/S2214-109X(21)00224-2, 29 July 2021)

EUPHA (2021). Statement on sexual and reproductive health and rights. (https://eupha.org/advocacy-by-eupha, 9 December 2021)

European Commission (2020). Gender Action Plan. Brussels: European Commission. (https://ec.europa.eu/international-partnerships/news/gender-action-plan-putting-women-and-girls-rights-heart-global-recovery-gender-equal-world_en, 16 June 2021)

European Commission (2021a). European Pillar of Social Rights Action Plan. Strasbourg: European Commission. (https://commission.europa.eu/publications/european-pillar-social-rights-action-plan_en)

European Commission (2021b). EUROSTAT. How has the EU progressed towards the Sustainable Development Goals? Brussels: European Commission. (https://ec.europa.eu/eurostat/web/products-eurostat-news/-/wdn-20210615-1, 17 June 2021)

European Network against Racism (2020). Why intersectionality is relevant for a fairer Europe. (https://www.enar-eu.org/Why-intersectionality-is-relevant-for-a-fairer-Europe, 12 July 2021)

European Parliament (2021). COVID-19 and its economic impact on women and women's poverty. Brussels, European Parliament's Policy Department for Citizens' Rights and Constitutional Affairs at the request of the FEMM Committee. (https://www.europarl.europa.eu/RegData/etudes/STUD/2021/693183/IPOL_STU(2021)693183_EN.pdf, 10 July 2021)

Fair F, Soltani H, Raben L et al. (2021). Midwives' experiences of cultural competency training and providing perinatal care for migrant women: a mixed methods study: Operational Refugee and Migrant Maternal Approach (ORAMMA) Project. BMC Pregnancy Childbirth, 21:340

GENCAD (2017). Gender differences in coronary artery disease in Europe. Brussels: European Union. (https://ec.europa.eu/health/sites/default/files/social_determinants/docs/2017_gencad_gendercoronaryarterydisease_flyer_en.pdf, 30 July 2021)

Global Health 50/50 (2021). The Sex, Gender and COVID-19 Health Policy Portal. (https://globalhealth5050.org/the-sex-gender-and-covid-19-project/policy-portal/, 16 June 2021)

Gofen A, Lotta G (2021). Street-level bureaucrats at the forefront of pandemic response: a comparative perspective. J Comp Policy Anal, 23:3–15.

Greer SL, Vasev N, Jarman H et al. (2019). It's the governance, stupid! TAPIC: A governance framework to strengthen decision making and implementation. Policy Brief 33. Copenhagen: European Observatory on Health Systems and Policies. (https://iris.who.int/handle/10665/331963)

Greer SL, King EJ, Massard da Fonseca E et al. (eds) (2021). Coronavirus Politics. The Comparative Politics and Policy of COVID-19. Ann Arbor, MI: University of Michigan Press. (https://doi.org/10.3998/mpub.11927713, 6 July 2021)

Gupta GR, Oomman N, Grown C et al. on behalf of the Gender Equality, Norms, and Health Steering Committee (2019). SDG5 Gender equality and gender norms: framing the opportunities for health. Lancet, 393:2550–2562.

Gupta N (2019). Research to support evidence-informed decisions on optimizing gender equity in health workforce policy and planning. Hum Resour Health, 17:46.

Haraway D (1988). Situated knowledges: the science question in feminism and the privilege of a partial perspective. Fem Stud, 14(3):575–599.

Hawkes S, Buse K (2013). Gender and global health: evidence, policy, and inconvenient truths. Lancet, 381:1783–1787.

Hulley S, Grady D, Bush T et al., for the Heart and Estrogen/progestin Replacement Study (HERS) Research Group (1998). Randomized trial of estrogenplus progestin for secondary prevention of coronary heart disease in postmenopausal women. JAMA, 280:605–613.

ILO (2020). A gender-responsive employment recovery: building back fairer. ILO Policy Brief. (https://www.ilo.org/emppolicy/pubs/WCMS_751785/lang–en/index.htm, 9 December 2021)

Krieger N, Davey Smith G (2004). Bodies count, and body counts: social epidemiology and embodying inequality. Epidemiol Rev, 26(1):92–103.

Kuhlmann E (2009). From women's health to gender mainstreaming and back again: linking feminist agendas and health policy. Curr Sociol, 57(2):135–154.

Kuhlmann E, Annandale E (2012). Mainstreaming gender into healthcare: a scoping exercise into policy transfer in England and Germany. Curr Sociol, 60(4):551–568.

Kuhlmann E, Annandale E (2015). Gender and healthcare policy. In: Kuhlmann E, Blank RH, Bourgeault I et al. (eds) The Palgrave International Handbook of Healthcare Policy and Governance. Basingstoke: Palgrave; 578–596.

Kuhlmann E, Ovseiko P, Kurmeyer C et al. (2017). Closing the gender leadership gap: a multi-centre cross-country comparison of women in management and leadership in academic health centres in the European Union. Hum Resour Health, 15:2.

Kuhlmann E, Lotta G, Fernandez M et al. (2023). SDG5 'Gender Equality' and the COVID-19 pandemic: a rapid assessment of health system responses in selected upper-middle and high-income countries. Front Public Health, 11:1078008. doi: 10.3389/fpubh.2023.1078008.

Lancet (2021). Editorial. COVID-19 in Latin America – emergency and opportunity. Lancet, 398:93.

Leppo K, Ollila E, Peña S et al. (2013). Health in All Policies. Seizing opportunities, implementing policies. Finland: Ministry of Social Affairs and Health.

Lotta G, Kuhlmann E (2021). When informal work and poor work conditions backfire and fuel the COVID-19 pandemic: why we should listen to the lessons from Latin America. Int J Health Plann Manage, 36:976–979.

Lotta G, Fernandez M, Pimenta D et al. (2021). Gender, race, and health workers in the COVID-19 pandemic. Lancet, 397(10281):1264. (https://doi.org/10.1016/S0140-6736(21)00530-4, 5 July 2021)

Lotta G, Fernandez M, Kuhlmann E et al. (2022). COVID-19 vaccination challenge: what have we learned from the Brazilian process? Lancet Global Health, 10(5):e613–e614. (https://doi.org/10.1016/S2214-109X(22)00049)

Lowy Institute (2021). Covid Performance Index. (https://interactives.lowyinstitute.org/features/covid-performance/, 7 July 2021).

McQueen DV, Wismar M, Lin V et al. (2012). Intersectoral governance for health in all policies: structures, actions and experiences. WHO Regional Office for Europe.

Morgan R, Baker P, Griffith DM et al. (2021). Beyond a zero-sum game: how does the impact of COVID-19 vary by gender? Front Sociol, 6. (https://www.frontiersin.org/articles/10.3389/fsoc.2021.650729/full, 5 July 2021)

ORAMMA Operational Refugee and Maternal Approach (2020). Layman Report, 2020. (http://oramma.eu/wp-content/uploads/2019/07/D2.2_layman-version.pdf, 16 June 2021)

ORAMMA Operational Refugee and Maternal Approach (n.d.). The project, without year. (http://oramma.eu/the-project/, 16 June 2021)

Ovseiko PV, Greenhalgh T, Adam P et al. (2017). A global call for action to include gender in research impact assessment. Health Res Policy Syst, 14:50.

Page E (2005). Joined-up government and the civil service. Joined-up government, 139–156.

Paine EA (2018). Embodied disruption: "Sorting out" gender and nonconformity in the doctor's office. Soc Sci Med, 211:352–358.

Petelos E, Vivilaki V, Papadakaki M et al. (2019). Training development in the ORAMMA (Operational Refugee and Migrant Maternal Approach) project. Eur J Public Health, 29(Supplement 4). DOI: 10.1093/eurpub/ckz186.049, 29 July 2021.

Rajan S, Richiardi W, McKee M (2020). The SDGs and health systems: the last step on the long and unfinished journey to universal health care? Eur J Public Health, 30(Suppl 1):i28–i31.

Rice S, Oliffe J, Seidler Z et al. (2021). Gender norms and the mental health of boys and young men. Lancet Public Health, 6:e541–e542.

Rocha R, Atun R, Massuda A et al. (2021). Effect of socioeconomic inequalities and vulnerabilities on health-system preparedness and response to COVID-19 in Brazil: a comprehensive analysis. Lancet, 9(6):e782–792. (https://doi.org/10.1016/S2214-109X(21)00081-4, 5 July 2021)

Sen G, Östlin P, George A (2007). Unequal, unfair, ineffective and inefficient. Gender inequity in health: why it exists and what we can do. Final report to the Women and Gender Equity Knowledge Network on the WHO Commission on Social Determinants of Health. Stockholm: Karolinska Institutet. (https://www.academia.edu/22882974/Women_and_Gender_Equity_Knowledge_Network, 28 July 2021)

Shamseer L, Bourgeault IL, Grunfeld E et al. (2021). Will COVID-19 result in a giant step backwards for women in academic science? J Clin Epidemiol, 134:160–166.

Spotlight Initiative to end violence against women and girls (2021). United Nations/European Commission. (https://spotlightinitiative.org/, 8 December 2021)

Takemoto MLS, McKay G, Amorim M et al. (2021). How can countries create outbreak response policies that are sensitive to maternal health? BMJ. (http://eprints.lse.ac.uk/110716/2/bmj.n1271.full.pdf, 5 July 2021)

Tomsick E, Smith J, Wenham C (2022). A gendered content analysis of the World Health Organization's COVID-19 guidance and policies. PLOS Glob Public Health, 2(6): e00006490. (https://doi.org/10.1371/journal.pgph.0000640)

UNDP-UN Women (2020). COVID-19 global gender response tracker, Global Fact Sheet. (https://www.undp.org/publications/covid-19-global-gender-response-tracker-fact-sheets, 29 July 2021)

United Nations (1999). Women and Health. Mainstreaming the Gender Perspective into the Health Sector. New York: UN Publication Sales No 99.IV.4.

Ventura D, Lotta G, Pereira C et al. (2021). Covid-19: Bolsonaro tells Brazilians to stop 'being a country of sissies'. BMJ Opinion. (https://blogs.bmj.com/bmj/2021/05/04/covid-19-bolsonaro-tells-brazilians-to-stop-being-a-country-of-sissies/, 29 July 2021).

Vijayasingham L, Bischof E, Wolfe J, on behalf of the Gender and COVID-19 Research Agenda-setting Initiative (2021). Sex-disaggregated data in COVID-19 vaccine trials. Lancet, 397(10278):966–967. (http://doi.org/10.1016/S0140-6736(21)00384-6, 30 July 2021)

Wenger NK (2012). Women and coronary heart disease: a century after Herrick. Understudied, underdiagnosed, and undertreated. Circulation, 126:604–611.

Wenham C (2021). Feminist Global Health Security. New York: Oxford University Press.

Wenham C, Smith J, Morgan R, on behalf of the Gender and COVID-19 Working Group (2020). COVID-19: the gendered impacts of the outbreak, Lancet, 395:846–848. (https://doi.org/10.1016/ S0140-6736(20)30526–2)

WHO (2002). WHO Multi-Country Study on Women's Health and Domestic Violence against Women. Geneva: World Health Organization. (https:// www.who.int/reproductivehealth/publications/violence/24159358X/en/, 29 July 2021)

WHO (2009). Strategy for integrating gender analysis and actions into the work of WHO. Geneva: World Health Organization. (https://www.who .int/publications/i/item/WHO-FCH-GWH-08.1, 19 August 2022)

WHO (2019). Framework for Action. Strengthening quality midwifery education for Universal Health Coverage 2030. Geneva: World Health Organization. (https://apps.who.int/iris/rest/bitstreams/1230352/retrieve, 9 December 2019)

WHO (2020a). COVID-19 and violence against women: what the health sector/system can do. Geneva: World Health Organization. (https://apps .who.int/iris/handle/10665/331699, 16 June 2021)

WHO (2020b). Gender and COVID-19 Advocacy Brief. Geneva: World Health Organization. (https://apps.who.int/iris/bitstream/ handle/10665/332080/WHO-2019-nCoV-Advocacy_brief-Gender-2020.1- eng.pdf?sequence=1&isAllowed=y, 16 June 2021)

WHO (2020c). Coronavirus disease (COVID-19) situation report 166. Geneva: World Health Organization. (https://www.who.int/docs/default- source/coronavirus/situation-reports/20200704-covid-19-sitrep-166 .pdf?sfvrsn=6247972_2, 29 July 2021)

WHO (2021). Working for better health for everyone, everywhere. Geneva: World Health Organization. (https://www.who.int/about/what-we-do/ who-brochure, 12 July 2021)

WHO Europe (2017). Fact sheets. Sustainable Development Goals: health targets. Sexual and Reproductive Health. Copenhagen: World Health Organization. (https://www.euro.who.int/__data/assets/pdf_ file/0005/348008/Fact-sheet-SDG-SRH-FINAL-04-09-2017.pdf, 4 July 2021)

WHO Europe (2018). Fact sheets. Sustainable Development Goals: health targets. Health Workforce. Copenhagen: World Health Organization. (https://www.euro.who.int/__data/assets/pdf_file/0004/381406/3.c- Worforce-Fact-sheet-eng.pdf, 4 July 2021)

Zuccala E, Horton ER (2018). Addressing the unfinished agenda on sexual and reproductive health and rights in the SDG era. Lancet, 391:2582–2583.

8 SDG8, promoting decent work and economic growth: health policies for good jobs

GEMMA A. WILLIAMS, OLIVIA A. ROCKWELL, SCOTT L. GREER

8.1 Introduction: what is SDG8 and how can health policy contribute?

Health is wealth. As the introductory chapters have shown, decent work and economic growth benefit greatly from a healthy population. However, the possible contribution of health policy to SDG8 goes beyond its contribution to population health because of the massive economic and employment footprint of health care and related systems. This chapter explores how health policy can help support progress towards SDG8 (creating decent work and economic growth), in light of the health and care sector being a major source of employment globally. Although health policy also contributes substantially to economic growth by improving the health and therefore productivity of the population, this is discussed elsewhere in this volume and is not covered in this chapter. We include a case study which explores health policy actions taken in Romania to improve attraction, recruitment and retention of health and care workers (HCWs). Romania is chosen as a case study as it highlights a number of common health and care workforce (HCWF) challenges experienced by countries globally. These include chronic shortages of HCWs that have been exacerbated by substantial outward migration, maldistribution in rural and remote areas, and insufficient skillmix to meet population health needs. With the health and care sector a major employer globally, efforts to strengthen the health workforce can support progress towards meeting SDG8. While not the primary focus of this chapter, it is important to note that actions to strengthen the HCWF can also help promote better health and wellbeing for all (SDG3) and better educational opportunities (SDG4). Moreover, positive outcomes related to employment and education are likely to especially benefit women

(SDG5), who are estimated to make up two-thirds of those employed in health and social care globally (Magar et al., 2016).

8.2 Background

SDG8 calls for countries to "promote sustained, inclusive and sustainable economic growth, full and productive employment and decent work for all". Health and long-term care and broader industries affected by health policy are major employers that can affect their own and others' labour market prospects. The HCWF is estimated to directly account for 3.4% of total global employment, ranging from 1% of total employment in low- and middle-income countries and up to 10% in high-income countries (WHO & ILO, 2022). Some industries related to health care, such as research, higher education and pharmaceuticals, are also important contributors to employment in many countries (see also Chapter 9).

Health and long-term care is a well known driver of employment growth. This is for a variety of reasons, but one is simply that it is a high-touch service sector that is difficult to make more efficient. Many consultations with health care professionals or contacts with social care workers are provided on a one-on-one basis, and making them handle more patients in a day is likely to reduce the quality of their work and comprehensiveness of their services. Even clearly efficiency-increasing options such as telehealth consultations can turn out to have potential and unpredictable quality and cost implications.

Thus, due to factors like an expanding sector, changing population demographics, and the necessity to maintain high standards of care, health and care sector employment tends to grow. This tendency for employment growth is known to economists as Baumol's disease (Baumol, 1967). While growth and industry change make cost containment difficult, it does mean that growing health systems increasingly make up a large portion of the economy, therefore becoming increasingly important employers across countries. Greater numbers of people thus depend on health care incomes and health care system employment standards. Consequently, this employment growth and subsequent power means that health and care employers will have a large impact on a substantial portion of employable individuals through health sector decisions, governance and overall wages.

The health and long-term care sector can also be an important potential contributor to reducing employment-related inequalities (see also Chapters 7 and 10). Health care providers are often geographically dispersed across diverse localities, which means that health employers might be one of the few, and amongst the most important, employers in poorer areas. Health care and related sectors also employ people at a wide range of skill levels, formal education and salaries, such as highly trained specialist doctors, home health aides, administrators, hospital porters and people without extensive educational credentialling. In addition, health care and related sectors in most countries employ a large number of women, migrants and minorities, shaping prospects for people across the society. (WHO & ILO, 2022).

Finally, health care is responsive to the state because of substantial public/parapublic funding and extensive regulation. While changing health systems and implementing even simple policies is notoriously difficult, there is still a variety of tools such as financing, regulation and professional standards that can be used by policymakers.

8.3   Causal pathways

Health policy can contribute to attainment of SDG8 through the health and care sector's role as a major employer (Fig. 8.1). SDG Target 8.2 calls for countries to achieve higher levels of economic productivity, in part by focusing on "high value-added and labor-intensive sectors". SDG Targets 8.5, 8.6 and 8.8, meanwhile, focus on reducing employment-related inequities for all women and men – including migrants, people living with disabilities and young people – by promoting full employment, decent work with equal pay for equal value, and safe and secure working environments.

As highlighted above, the health and care sector is highly labour-intensive as well as being a major employer of women, migrants and young people globally. Health sectors can therefore play a key role in meeting SDG targets of promoting decent jobs and reducing employment-related inequalities, consequently driving productivity and economic growth. The co-benefits are both direct, through the impact of health employment on employees, and indirect, through the impact of the health sector's actions on the broader labour market.

Indirectly, health policy can affect local and national economies because of the size and diversity of the HCWF. In local labour markets

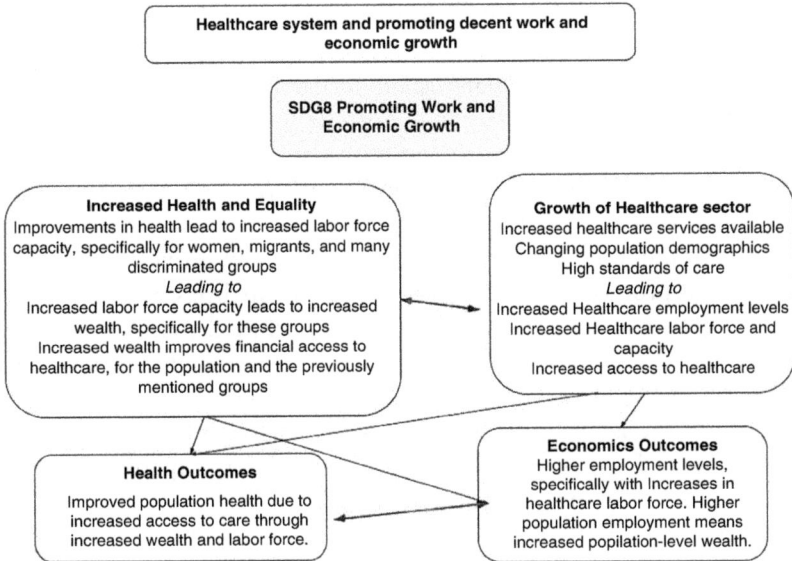

Fig. 8.1 Causal pathway mapping for SDG8: the health and economic outcomes, as influenced by governance mechanisms used by the combined economic and health sectors

they can influence overall wage-setting and employment conditions, both as a workforce model and by competing with other businesses for talented staff. Unionization also typically builds outward from areas of labour strength, so a unionized health care sector can be a linchpin for broader and potentially beneficial social partnership. Moreover, the health sector indirectly has a significant multiplier effect on the overall labour force and economy, by creating and supporting jobs in industries that drive innovation such as in pharmaceuticals, digital health technologies, research and development, and manufacturing (for example, medical equipment, physical infrastructure, etc.). While there is limited evidence on multiplier effects in low- and middle-income countries, multiplier effects in high-income countries are substantial. In Spain, for example, the health technology industry employed 28 500 people in 2020 and generated a turnover of €8.8 billion (Bernal-Delgado & Al Tayara, 2022). In France, digital health start-ups were estimated to have an annual turnover of €800 million in 2019, rising to a projected €40 billion by 2030, while the medical devices sector had a turnover of €30 billion in 2019 and generated 90 000 jobs (Or & Al Tayara, 2022). Given that health and care and related industries are both high value added and labour-intensive, the surrounding industries not only have inherent value but also can contribute to the broader attainment of SDG8's goal of decent work and economic growth.

Directly, the functions within an employment system of hiring, pay, job design and career paths of health and care-related employers can contribute to reducing various inequalities and provide good jobs. Hiring and promotion systems can reduce inequalities by eliminating discriminatory practices that lead to less well-paid jobs for women, people with disabilities and other racial, religious and ethnic minorities. Reducing discriminatory pay differentials within jobs and discriminatory job classifications (for example, putting women into job categories with lower pay and worse prospects) can contribute to equality. Having standardized working conditions, transparent pay scales, formalizing informal jobs – particularly in long-term care – and tackling negative stereotypes around marginalized groups can further help promote equality. Other tasks that can use health policy to help reduce employment-related inequalities can be as distinctive as diversifying medical school admissions and hiring in order to have doctors who better represent the population at large, creating permanent and stable positions for traditionally precarious workforces in areas such as care for older people. Developing coherent career paths and equal opportunities for further training and promotion can enable upward mobility within organizations for those who might find fewer opportunities to rise in the broader economy.

All of this will have an impact on education, as to train a workforce that empowers and enables those historically overlooked will entail equal educational opportunities for all individuals (SDG4). Efforts to promote equal opportunities necessarily need to start early, by encouraging women and ethnic minorities to consider careers in STEM (science, technology, engineering and mathematics) (WHO & ILO, 2022).

Creating decent work for all relies on creating conditions that promote a healthy work environment, a good work-life balance, and stable and fair employment conditions. Some effective health policy instruments to achieve these aims include ensuring fair remuneration, flexible working, safe staffing levels, limits on working hours, providing childcare and improving workplace occupational health and safety, among others (WHO Regional Office for Europe, 2022). Creating and maintaining systems and policies that promote training and promotion paths and offering lifelong training are also important to allow employees upward occupational mobility if desired.

Overall, there are vast opportunities to use health policy to create employment and decent work for all within the health and care sector, and a substantial body of literature on education and management exists that proposes and tests interventions and policy ideas. However, these policy options are often not used effectively or at all, and many inefficiencies continue to persist in relation to the health and workforce globally. For example, it has been estimated that worldwide women wage earners in the health and care sector earn almost 20% less than men, with women overrepresented in lower paid occupational categories and men in higher paid occupational categories (WHO & ILO, 2022). Moreover, many countries are experiencing major shortages of HCWs and have insufficient skillmix to meet population health needs. In part, this is due to failures to enhance attraction, recruitment and retention of HCWs by improving employment and working conditions, including remuneration and career opportunities. Failure to address these inefficiencies in the HCWF will not only undermine efforts to meet SDG8 but will curb progress towards universal health coverage and achieving good health and wellbeing for all (SDG3).

8.4 Governance and politics: conceptual issues

Governance is how societies make and implement decisions. The contribution of health policy to most SDGs requires a great deal of intersectoral collaboration and governance. This is also the case for SDG8. Ensuring the sustainable supply and employment of HCWs requires the health and care sector to work together with other sectors, including the education, labour and finance sectors, although this is not always achieved in practice. A range of cross-sectoral governance actions, such as regulating and accrediting educational institutions, policies on access to the health labour market and setting general conditions of work and employment, all play a key role in shaping the HCWF (WHO Regional Office for Europe, 2022). Furthermore, departments of social protection and social affairs can play a key role in developing polices to reduce horizontal and vertical gender segregation (WHO Regional Office for Europe, 2022).

Matching and maximizing the contribution of health policy to SDG8 nevertheless primarily requires changes within the health sector. Health policymakers generally have access to key policy tools for improving employment and working conditions: sectoral bargaining systems, labour contracts, regulatory and inspection standards, accreditation and credentialling, and civil service rules. The governance of the health sector is what matters, including the range of available policy tools and rules for making decisions. The involvement and influence of the state, however, vary considerably between countries. A centralized national health service, for example, may generally have a larger regulatory and enforcement role than a fragmented health service with a large private sector, where regulation and enforcement might be difficult or not feasible.

The politics of attaining SDG8 through health are challenging because they frequently involve additional costs. Workplace health and safety measures will often have immediate and visible costs (equipment, slower working) even if they lead to longer-term benefits by reducing injuries, promoting mental health and ensuring quality and safety. Efforts to improve hostile workplace climates (for example, by addressing bullying or sexual abuse) can be difficult and may alienate powerful people who enjoy, and might have created, that climate. More equal pay and conditions will require either additional funds, redistribution from other health care budget areas or redistribution of expenditure away from the best-paid towards the worst-paid – for example, from the clinical workforce to the non-clinical workforce. In turn, this means confronting entrenched interests and, in many cases, constraints imposed by cost containment. Those entrenched interests can include unions and incumbent employees with strong legal protections if they do not feel that they or their members would benefit from changing employment conditions (a problem of labour market dualism that can entrench inequality between protected workers in unionized positions and unprotected workers without unions). They can also include outsourcing firms. In many cases, services that employ many workers who are the victims of discrimination, such as facilities maintenance and home health care, are outsourced to private firms to reduce costs. With private health care providers profit-focused, they are often unwilling to improve their workers' salaries and working conditions. The employees might be both precarious and invisible to health policymakers, but the employers are likely to be well organized and politically represented. Finally, the effects of spending more in health affects other public employees and might create pressure to increase salaries in other sectors.

There are also strong arguments to be made against being a better employer than is strictly necessary. Efficiency can appear to be improved in many cases if there are fewer employees, they have more work, or their workplace does not adhere to the highest standards of health and safety. Why should (often publicly financed) systems pay more than they must to recruit staff?

Against this way of thinking, it is clear that there are long-run benefits to being a better employer. This is the basis of the economic concept of the "efficiency wage" (Akerlof, 1984; Akerlof & Yellen, 1986). Above-market wages are paid to improve productivity and reduce the rates of sick leave by having a happier, more stable workforce that requires less oversight, can be trained to higher levels, and is not subject to all the cost and quality problems associated with turnover.

In many cases, the result is that healthcare workforce becomes a low-salience, high-conflict area of policy, wherein policymakers have limited incentive to start politically unrewarding arguments about expensive policies with professionals, unions, companies or managers. Politically, then, who can raise the salience of the issues incorporated in SDG8 and perhaps formulate solutions that gain agreement? The clearest answer is organizations that represent the groups who stand to benefit the most: unions, civil society organizations and advocates representing women, workers and minority groups who are the subject of discrimination. Broader coalitions in support of health policies that support SDG8 might include local governments, patient and community groups, and professional organizations. Publicized scandals (such as deaths among care workers and the older people they served during the COVID-19 pandemic) can sometimes lead to change.

It will always be difficult to avoid conflict when the subject is pay and conditions of publicly financed work, but increased budgets can ease distributive conflicts. It is not an accident that Agenda for Change, which regraded and shifted pay scales across the English NHS, happened at a time of substantial budget increases. These public budget increases meant that differentials at the bottom could be reduced while still increasing pay at the top of the income scale. Times and circumstances, like those created by the Agenda for Change, of increased health expenditure create an agreeable environment in which to push health systems towards supporting the goals of SDG8.

8.5   Country case study: tackling health worker shortages and maldistribution in Romania

As demonstrated, the health sector can play a key role in promoting economic growth, employment and decent work for all. Maximizing the contribution of the health sector to SDG8 nevertheless requires policy actions to ensure a sufficient supply, efficient employment, and equal geographic distribution of HCWs. In this case study, we provide an overview of policy actions taken in Romania to address health workforce shortages and other workforce deficiencies such as insufficient skillmix, by tackling issues related to recruitment, retention, maldistribution and international mobility of health workers. While Romania has experienced chronic health workforce shortages since the 1990s, this case study focuses on recent policy actions that were undertaken to address a substantial increase in outward migration of health workers after the country's accession to the EU in 2007. It should be noted that the recent, or in some cases ongoing, implementation of these reforms means that their full impact cannot yet be assessed.

8.5.1   *Romania has a chronic shortage and insufficient skillmix of health and long-term care workers especially in rural and deprived areas*

Romania has a highly centralized, Social Health Insurance-based health system. Health spending increased by approximately 10.3% annually between 2015 and 2019 but remains among the lowest in the EU when measured as a share of GDP (5.7% in 2019) or per capita (EUR) (OECD & European Observatory on Health Systems and Policies, 2021). The health sector in Romania accounted for approximately 5% of the economically active population (over 15 years of age) in 2018, making it an important source of employment in the country (Eurostat, 2020). The country has nevertheless faced long-standing issues over health worker shortages, in particular in rural and deprived areas. The number of practising physicians per capita (3.1 per 1000 population) in 2018 was the third lowest in the EU. The number of nurses (7.2 per 1000) was also below the EU average (8.2 per 1000) (OECD.stat, 2021). Alongside a shortage of GPs, the COVID-19 pandemic has highlighted acute shortages among intensive care unit (ICU) physicians, nurses and other specialized health care staff and carers. Persistent health worker shortages and maldistribution have contributed to geographic disparities in access to care and inequalities in health outcomes for vulnerable groups, and have had a deleterious impact on quality of care (OECD & European Observatory on Health Systems and Policies, 2021; Vlădescu et al., 2016).

Prominent causes of health and long-term care worker shortages in Romania include low salaries compared to other sectors, limited career development opportunities, poor working conditions, a gap between required competencies and working opportunities – partly due to lack of modern technologies – and insufficient recognition and social status (Galan, Olsavszky & Vlădescu, 2011). Workforce challenges were further exacerbated by responses to the economic crisis in 2009/10, which saw budget constraints placed on hospitals' staffing capacity and a recruitment freeze and salary cut of 25% introduced in the public sector (Suciu et al., 2017).

These issues have seen young people increasingly opt for more attractive careers in other sectors, while a significant number of health professionals have left the public sector or migrated abroad (Vlădescu et al., 2016). The challenge of outward migration increased dramatically after 2007, when EU accession and the associated rights of free movement and mutual recognition of qualifications provided new opportunities to seek better remuneration, working conditions and training opportunities in other countries. While accurate data on migration trends are limited for most professions, it is estimated that from 2007 to 2013 approximately 14 000 physicians left to work abroad[1] (Paina, Ungureanu & Olsavszky, 2016), with France, Germany and the UK popular countries of destination (Williams et al., 2020). In the long-term care sector, the exact number of carers who have migrated is unknown due to the scarcity of data.

8.5.2 Tackling health worker shortages in Romania is a political priority

Addressing shortages and maldistribution of health workers has become a political priority in Romania owing to concerns over the impact on health and quality of care. Accordingly, an objective was included in the "National Health Strategy 2014–2020: Health for Prosperity", to implement sustainable human resources for health strategy. A National

---

[1] To place this in context, Romania had an estimated 39 000 registered physicians in 2014 (Paina, Ungureanu & Olsavszky, 2016).

Action Plan for Human Resources was later developed in 2016, with agreement from policymakers, labour unions and professional associations. The primary aims are to strengthen health workforce governance, data flows and research evidence to improve planning and policymaking (Ungureanu & Socha-Dietrich, 2019). A Human Resources for Health Centre was also created in 2017 by the Ministry of Health to improve planning and management for the medical workforce and to support the return of physicians who have migrated. A national registry of health professionals in the country is currently under development (Ungureanu & Socha-Dietrich, 2019).

The Romanian government has also taken on responsibility for improving the professional status of health workers by increasing salaries and developing performance assessment criteria and career pathways. As part of the vision for the Government Programme 2017–2022, a "motivating salary package" for health professionals was included as a key reform to reduce the number leaving the public health workforce (Scîntee & Vlădescu, 2018). Alongside addressing low salaries, these reforms also explicitly aimed to boost employment and the economy. The Committees for Labour and Social Protections, and Budget, Finance and Banks within the Chamber of Deputies approved small salary increases for health professionals in 2016, with commitments for further increases and improvements to working conditions by 2022 (Law 153/2017). While the vision to raise salaries gained broad political support and was seen as justified, it created some political conflict with the opposition party. The criticism pointed to a significant increase in Romania's budget deficit, ultimately undermining the country's fiscal sustainability. This would be especially true if other public sector workers asked for a salary increase (Table 8.1).

Table 8.1 *Political importance and conflict: the context of policymaking and implementation of reforms to increase health worker salaries*

| | | Conflict | | |
		Low	Medium	High
Political importance	High		x	
	Medium			
	Low			

The limited initial increase in salaries and the phased approach to improvement were not deemed acceptable by health professionals and their trade unions, leading to protest rallies and strikes supported by the public (Scîntee & Vlădescu, 2018). Successful negotiations between the government and representatives of health workers ultimately led the government to amend Law 153/2017 through an Emergency Ordinance in December 2017 to bring forward salary increases for physicians, nurses and other health workers in the public sector from 1 March 2018 (Scîntee & Vlădescu, 2018). Upon implementation, the average salary of a junior doctor increased by approximately 162%, and the average salary of a senior physician by 131%. While data on the impact of this reform are not yet available, the Ministry of Health has suggested there are early signs of more Romanian physicians expressing an interest in returning home to practise (Scîntee & Vlădescu, 2018). Nevertheless, the reform only targeted hospital-based doctors and has not addressed low salaries for GPs, which may contribute to a weakening of primary care and exacerbate inefficiencies in the health system in the future.

Other efforts to boost recruitment and retention of health professionals and to enhance skillmix include strategies to improve career development opportunities and working conditions. For example, specialization options for nurses have also been expanded through Order 942/2017, to include new disciplines such as paediatrics, psychiatry, oncology and community care, among others (Vlădescu & Scîntee, 2017). The Ministry of Health also took steps to reform residency options for medical graduates to reduce physician shortages in rural areas and for certain specialties. Under the reforms, graduates must work in a particular location or a particular specialty with shortages for the time of their medical training. However, while formal evaluations have not been conducted, some preliminary evidence suggests that poor management and lack of enforcement of contracts has seen a high proportion of residents dropping out of residencies early (Paina, Ungureanu & Olsavszky, 2016; Ungureanu & Socha-Dietrich, 2019).

8.5.3 Responding to health worker shortages requires international initiatives and cooperation

International actors have also played an important role in helping to strengthen Romania's HCWF. In particular, the EU has launched a number of initiatives to help Member States improve workforce planning, training, development and retention. For example, a number of measures have been implemented with support from European and Structural Investment Funds (ESIF) to: increase competencies in certain medical practices such as minimally invasive surgeries, oncology and endocrinology; provide more training opportunities; enhance digital capacities; and increase access to modern equipment (OECD & European Observatory on Health Systems and Policies, 2021). The EU's Recovery and Resilience Facility initiated in 2021 in response to the COVID-19 pandemic has also provided funding that can be used to improve education systems and skills of health workers (Williams et al., 2022). Under this initiative, Romania's Recovery and Resilience plan has been granted funding to improve "capacity for health management and human resources in health". Specific measures that will be taken to meet this objective include the preparation of the Strategy for Human Resources Development for 2022–2030, training for health workers, and the establishment of the National Institute for Health Services Management (Scîntee & Vlădescu, 2022).

International cooperation and initiatives have also been put in place to help manage the international migration of health workers. A significant global effort in this area includes the development and adoption by WHO Member States in 2010 of the "WHO Global Code of Practice on the International Recruitment of Health Personnel" (WHO, 2010). The Global Code established "voluntary principles and practices" to reduce active recruitment of health workers from low- and middle-income countries facing critical shortages, while encouraging countries to strengthen their domestic workforces (WHO, 2010). To support monitoring of the Code in Europe, the OECD, WHO-Europe and EUROSTAT have worked together to extend data collection on health worker mobility to the entire region. It is important to note that the Code recognizes that international migration can be of benefit for source and destination countries if managed properly, for example, through the use of bilateral country agreements (Williams et al., 2020). Romania itself has signed 11 bilateral agreements, although many of these pre-date the existence of the Code (for example, with Germany in 2005 to manage the recruitment of nursing aides). The impact of these bilateral agreements overall has not been monitored, making their effectiveness unknown.

8.5.4 Multiple intersectoral governance structures and governance actions have been used to respond to health worker shortages

Ministerial linkages and stakeholder engagement across government ministries and with professional associations, trade unions and health professionals themselves have been key drivers of reforms at the national level (Table 8.2). Governance actions from the government and Ministry of Health have involved setting targets and goals, developing policies and strategies, and proving a legal mandate and financial support

Table 8.2 *Governance actions and intersectoral structures driving health workforce reforms*

Tools			Possible governance actions with these tools								
			Goals and targets	Evidence support	Policy guidance	Implementation and management	Coordination	Advocacy	Monitoring and evaluation	Financial support	Legal mandate
	Plan	Plan									
	Indicators and Targets	Indicators									
		Targets									
	Budgeting	European and Structural Investment Funds (ESIF)								x	x
		EU Recovery and Resilience Facility	x		x					x	
		Romania's Recovery and Resilience Facility	x							x	

Table 8.2 *(Cont.)*

		Possible governance actions with these tools								
Tools	**Organization**	Ministry of Health	x				x			x	x
		National Institute for Health Services Management				x	x				
		Trade Unions						x			x
		Health Professional Advocacy Groups						x			
	Accountability	WHO Global Code of Practice on the International Recruitment of Health Personnel	x	x				x			
		Independent agency/ evaluators									
		Human Resources for Health Centre				x	x		x		
		Support for civil society			x			x			x
		Legal rights									

for reforms. In addition, advocacy from health professionals and their representatives has played a key role in driving actions around salary increases and improvements to working conditions. International cooperation and coordination among key stakeholders including the WHO, the EU and major destination countries, along with EU funding, have also been critical to tackling the international mobility of health workers.

8.5.5　Romania has implemented a wide range of actions to tackle HCWF issues, but more remains to be done

Romania has taken a number of steps to address health workforce deficiencies. These actions have contributed to the number of physicians and nurses per capita working in the public sector increasing by 29% and 24% respectively since 2007 (OECD.stat, 2021). However, the density of doctors and nurses still remains among the lowest in the EU, and tackling overall shortages, maldistribution and insufficient skillmix continues to be of high political importance.

The HCWF challenges faced by Romania are not unique and are being experienced by countries worldwide. These issues are likely to become more severe in the aftermath of the COVID-19 pandemic, which has proved enormously challenging for health and care workers and led to a backlog of missed care in many countries (van Ginneken et al., 2022; Williams et al., 2022). Sustained action is therefore needed to strengthen the HCWF to ensure it can meet population health needs and respond to future emergencies. Improving salaries, working conditions, training opportunities and the development of competencies, along with joint workforce planning underpinned by better health workforce data, are some health policy areas that can contribute to meeting this aim and the objectives of SDG8 – decent work for all and economic growth.

8.6 Conclusion

Better health promotes better work and employment. Health policy itself can also promote better work and employment by improving health system standards and making health sector actors better employers. In many cases, these improvements involve redirecting or increasing health expenditure to improve the safety, quality and career progression of jobs at the lower ranks of the health system. Increasing public budgets can lead to political discourse when budgets already face constraints. However, if implemented well, changes in health expenditure can have benefits to the organization. A suggested solution includes paying an efficiency wage for better productivity rather than simply hiring at the lowest possible wage.

The governance mechanisms and tools are often already available in human resources policies and planning; thus, less innovation is required than is described in some other chapters of this book. Opportunities to improve workplaces are everywhere, from addressing certain management behaviours in particular units, to strong and well enforced antidiscrimination law, to paying a higher minimum wage, and schemes such as "Workers can be Allies". But the political difficulty is that, outside a large influx of funds, improving the quality of jobs and reducing inequalities will impose costs on organizations (for safer work, for adapting hiring procedures to not discriminate) and reduce pay differentials that benefit higher paid workers. The benefits to organizations of high-quality jobs without discrimination have not always convinced managers and policymakers. Focusing attention on political actors such as unions and civil society that will support SDG8 is therefore crucial.

References

Akerlof GA (1984). Gift exchange and efficiency-wage theory: Four views. Am Econ Rev, 74(2):79–83.

Akerlof GA, Yellen JL (eds) (1986). Efficiency wage models of the labor market. Cambridge: Cambridge University Press.

Baumol WJ (1967). Macroeconomics of unbalanced growth: the anatomy of urban crisis. Am Econ Rev, 57(3):415–426.

Bernal-Delgado E, Al Tayara L (2022). How does Spain's health sector contribute to the economy? Health and the Economy: A series of country snapshots. Copenhagen: WHO Regional Office for Europe on behalf of the European Observatory on Health Systems and Policies

Eurostat (2020). Majority of health jobs held by women. European Commission. (https://ec.europa.eu/eurostat/web/products-eurostat-news/-/DDN-20200409-2, 15 May 2021)

Galan A, Olsavszky V, Vladescu C (2011). Emergent challenge of health professional emigration: Romania's accession to the EU. In: Wismar M, Maier C, Glinos I et al. (eds) Health Professional Mobility and Health Systems. Evidence from 17 European Countries. WHO Regional Office for Europe on behalf of the European Observatory on Health Systems and Policies.

Magar V, Gerecke M, Dhillon I et al. (2016). Women's contributions to sustainable development through work in health: using a gender lens to advance a transformative 2030 agenda. In: Buchan J, Dhillon I, Campbell J (eds) Health employment and economic growth: an evidence base. Geneva: World Health Organization.

OECD.stat (2021). Health Care Resources. OECD statistics. (https://stats.oecd.org)

OECD/European Observatory on Health Systems and Policies (2021). Romania: Country Health Profile 2019. State of Health in the EU. Paris: OECD Publishing/Brussels: European Observatory on Health Systems and Policies.

Or Z, Al Tayara L (2022). How does France's Health Sector Contribute to the Economy? Health and the Economy: A series of country snapshots. WHO Regional Office for Europe.

Paina L, Ungureanu M, Olsavszky V (2016). Implementing the Code of Practice on International Recruitment in Romania—exploring the current state of implementation and what Romania is doing to retain its domestic health workforce. Hum Resour Health, 14(Suppl 1):22.

Scîntee G, Vlădescu C (2018). Update on measures to alleviate the shortage of human resources in the Romanian health system. Health Systems and Policy Monitor. European Observatory on Health Systems and Policies. (https://www.hspm.org/countries/romania23092016/livinghit.aspx?Section=4.1%20Regulation&Type=Chapter#10MeasurestobringbackRomaniandoctorsfromabroad)

Scîntee SG, Vlădescu C (2022). Increasing capacity for health management and human resources in health. Health System and Policy Monitor Country Update. European Observatory on Health Systems and Policies. (https://eurohealthobservatory.who.int/monitors/health-systems-monitor/analyses/hspm/romania-2016/increasing-capacity-for-health-management-and-human-resources-in-health)

Suciu ŞM, Popescu CA, Ciumageanu MD et al. (2017). Physician migration at its roots: a study on the emigration preferences and plans among medical students in Romania. Hum Resour Health, 15(6). (https://doi.org/10.1186/s12960-017-0181-8)

Ungureanu M, Socha-Dietrich K (2019). Romania: A growing international medical education hub. In: Recent Trends in International Migration of Doctors, Nurses and Medical Students. Paris: OECD.

van Ginneken E, Reed S, Siciliani L et al. (2022). Addressing backlogs and managing waiting lists during and beyond the COVID-19 pandemic. WHO Regional Office for Europe. (https://apps.who.int/iris/handle/10665/358832)

Vlădescu C, Scîntee SG (2017). Update on more specialization opportunities for nurses. Health Systems and Policy Monitor. European Observatory on Health Systems and Policies. (https://www.hspm.org/countries/romania23092016/livinghit.aspx?Section=4.1%20Regulation&Type=Chapter#10MeasurestobringbackRomaniandoctorsfromabroad)

Vlădescu C, Scîntee SG, Olsavszky V et al. (2016). Romania Health system review. Health Systems in Transition 18(4):1170. (https://www.euro.who.int/__data/assets/pdf_file/0017/317240/Hit-Romania.pdf, 16 June 2021)

WHO (2010). WHO Global Code of Practice on the International Recruitment of Health Personnel. Geneva: World Health Organization.

WHO, ILO (2022). The gender pay gap in the health and care sector: a global analysis in the time of COVID-19. (https://www.ilo.org/wcmsp5/groups/public/---dgreports/---dcomm/---publ/documents/publication/wcms_850909.pdf)

WHO Regional Office for Europe (2022). Health and care workforce in Europe: time to act. (https://www.who.int/europe/publications/i/item/9789289058339)

Williams GA, Jacob G, Rakovac I et al. (2020). Health professional mobility in the WHO European Region and the WHO Global Code of Practice: data from the joint OECD/ EUROSTAT/WHO-Europe questionnaire. Eur J Public Health, 30 (Suppl 4):iv5–iv11.

Williams GA, Maier CB, Scarpetti G et al. (2022). Human Resources for health during COVID-19: creating surge capacity and rethinking skill mix. Eurohealth; 28(1). (https://eurohealthobservatory.who.int/publications/i/health-system-resilience-post-covid-moving-towards-more-european-cooperation-(eurohealth))

9 SDG9, industry, innovation and infrastructure: technology and knowledge transfer as means to generate co-benefits between health and industrial Sustainable Development Goals

ELIZE MASSARD DA FONSECA, HELENA DE MORAES ACHCAR

9.1 Introduction

Ensuring universal health coverage requires a stable, affordable supply of drugs and vaccines. The current COVID-19 pandemic has exacerbated the need for low- and middle-income countries (LMICs) to strengthen (or build) their own health industrial capabilities that would allow them to gain a steady supply of vaccines and achieve faster immunization coverage. This chapter explores the links between Sustainable Development Goal 3 (SDG3) (specifically Targets 3.3, 3.8 and 3b, which address the need to fight communicable diseases, achieve universal health coverage, and invest in research and development of vaccines and medicines, respectively) and SDG9, which calls for the development of industry, innovation and infrastructure in LMICs. It argues that initiatives such as technology transfer and local production of pharmaceuticals in LMICs can be a means to promote industrial and innovation goals (for example, skills development and manufactory capacity-building), while meeting health needs.

The first parts of this chapter revisit the international commitments to align health and industrial goals and identify their causal pathways and limitations. Sections 9.4 and 9.5 present two case studies: 1) Brazil's technology transfer strategy for the human papillomavirus (HPV) vaccine through a public–private partnership between Merck Sharp & Dohme (MSD) and the Butantan Institute, a local, state-owned laboratory, and 2) the implementation of the *Sociedade Moçambicana de Medicamentos* (SMM, or Mozambican Pharmaceutical Ltd), a Brazil–Mozambique South–South cooperation (SSC) project for the implementation of an antiretroviral and other essential medications factory in this sub-Saharan African country.

Brazil has been known for integrating health and industrial policy through initiatives that foster technological development of local pharmaceutical companies through public–private partnerships (termed productive development partnerships, PDPs) (Flynn, 2015; Shadlen & Fonseca, 2013), and as such, the country merits attention. Brazil's successful domestic experience has also inspired the development of pharmaceutical technology and capacity-building in sub-Saharan Africa (Mackintosh et al., 2016).

Both cases illustrate the intersectoral initiatives between health and industrial policies in Brazil and Mozambique and how they have led to increased health benefits – such as sustainable and affordable access to the HPV vaccine in Brazil and essential medications in Mozambique – but also the industrial and technological co-benefits – such as the modernization of local state-owned laboratories and enhancement of technological and human capacity in both countries. Additionally, the cases illustrate co-benefits concerning other SDGs related to gender (SDG5 and SDG10), as well as cross-sector and cross-country collaboration.

The two case studies have significant variations between them, namely the fact that Brazil is an upper-middle-income country and Mozambique a low-income country. As such, these cases allow us to explore the dynamic interaction and co-benefits between SDG3 and SDG9 in different contexts and to study the complexities and difficulties as functions of these contexts. Although the two case studies can help elucidate the co-benefits between health policy and measures to promote scientific and technological development, further research is still needed to better understand which channels, governance arrangements, and mechanisms can promote effective coordination between the two sectors. Our analysis does not intend to be exhaustive in the possibilities and avenues for promoting co-benefits between SDG3 and SDG9. Also, although we focus primarily on the health care aspect of SDG3, the analyses presented in our chapter can stimulate investigation into other elements of public health, for instance, disease prevention (for example, the production of diagnostic test kits).

9.2 Background

This section briefly characterizes SDG9, its relevance to SDG3, and why it matters for co-benefits. SDG9 relates to three core aspects of sustainable development: infrastructure, industrialization and innovation. According to the first SDG progress report,

> Infrastructure provides the basic physical systems and structures essential to the operation of a society or enterprise. Industrialization drives economic growth, creates job opportunities and thereby reduces income poverty. Innovation advances the technological capabilities of industrial sectors and prompts the development of new skills. (United Nations Economic and Social Council, 2016, p. 13)

SDG9 has eight targets, which refer to "outcome targets" (such as upgrade all industries and infrastructures for sustainability, enhance research and upgrade industrial technologies) and "means of achieving targets" (such as facilitate sustainable infrastructure development for LMICs, and support domestic technology development and industrial diversification). The case of pharmaceutical technology transfer speaks well to these SDG9 targets as it requires building new infrastructure, it relates to a global industrial sector, and it is also innovative as it means gaining knowledge. Other areas of investigation would be medical technologies and devices, such as the surge of wearables to monitor people's health.

SDG9 is usually discussed in relation to environmental issues (Kynčlová, Upadhyaya & Nice, 2020). However, there are important synergies between SDG3 and SDG9, particularly Target 3b, which relates to the research and development of vaccines and medicines for the communicable and non-communicable diseases that primarily affect LMICs, as we shall see now.

One of the important societal challenges of our time is securing steady and affordable access to, and stimulating the development of, innovative health technologies in LMICs. In the early 2000s, the linkages between intellectual property regulation and access to biomedical technologies in LMICs became more evident and revealed the need for a new way of thinking about research and development (R&D) policies to respond to societal needs and demands. It was in this context, in 2008, that the World Health Assembly launched the Global Strategy and

Plan of Action on Public Health, Innovation and Intellectual Property (GSPA-PHI) (World Health Assembly, 2008). This plan represented not just a framework for action but also a fundamental paradigm shift for global R&D by focusing on priority diseases in LMICs (Nunn, Fonseca & Gruskin, 2009). For the first time, there was a global commitment to creating, and consensus on the need for, new mechanisms to incentivize R&D and the capacity to generate health innovations in LMICs. Today, although the linkages between health systems, innovation and health industry policies have become more visible (Natera, Tomassini & Vera-Cruz, 2019; Proksch et al., 2019), there is still a great need to explore the governance arrangements that connect these policies and their co-benefits.

Local pharmaceutical production and technology transfer were identified as means of bridging gaps in access to medicines and contributing to local economies in LMICs (Mackintosh et al., 2016; Russo & Banda, 2015; Shadlen & Fonseca, 2013). Throughout the years, the World Health Organization has developed an initiative to assist LMICs in strengthening their capacity to produce medicines (WHO, 2011). It also became clear that the limitations of the GSPA-PHI in promoting such initiatives as its goals were too broad for effective implementation (WHO, 2018).

The COVID-19 pandemic renewed the interest in technology transfer and local production of pharmaceuticals because of the need to scale up vaccine production to secure a stable supply and the challenges of ensuring equitable access to COVID-19 vaccines. In June 2021, the WHO organized the first World Local Production Forum (WLPF). The Forum aimed to call "Member States' attention in aligning the production of health products as essential long-term infrastructure akin to food, water and energy as safeguards to protect national, regional and global security" (WHO, 2021b). Therefore, the WHO recognizes that increasing investment in industrial development alone is not sufficient. It is the dynamic interaction of both realms, R&D and health systems, that matters (Santiago, 2020). Such intersectoral action cannot be built quickly during the pandemic era. It requires long-term investments to build partnerships and business linkages and develop knowledge in strategic sectors for national security – knowledge that can be applied during public health emergencies.

For instance, bridging health and industrial goals requires patent licences, strengthening the regulatory system, and building an ecosystem for local production, among other factors (WHO, 2021b). An ecosystem for local pharmaceutical production includes engagement of the trade, finance and judicial sectors of governments (WHO, 2021a). For instance, low access to capital is a key limiting factor for local manufacturers in LMICs; this requires long-term financial support from development banks and other financial institutions. According to the WHO, these elements would hopefully stimulate the development and sustainability of vibrant health product manufacturing industries in LMICs.

9.3 Causal pathways between health action and SDG9 co-benefits

There are actions that have the potential to build co-benefits between the health care sector and industry. One is the notion of PDPs. Initiatives such as the Drugs for Neglected Diseases initiative (DNDi) – which aimed at conducting and coordinating R&D for new drugs, diagnostics or vaccines – address pressing health needs in resource-limited settings. By doing so, since the early 2000s, DNDi has contributed to building innovation ecosystems in LMICs and invested in improving health infrastructure through clinic and laboratory renovations, the provision of essential equipment and supplies, and the continuous training of health personnel, with almost 5,000 people trained since 2010 in the Lead Optimization Latin America project[1] alone (Drugs for Neglected Diseases initiative, 2019).

Although our analysis focuses primarily on the LMICs context, experiences in industrialized nations illustrate the potential for generalizing our rationale of co-benefits between SDG3 and SDG9. For instance, promising actions are mission-driven innovation policies, which have been encouraged mainly by the European Commission (EU) (Directorate-General for Research and Innovation, 2003; Kok, 2004).[2] For instance, the EU Horizon 2020 research and innovation programme (2014–2020) aimed to combine solutions to broad societal challenges as drivers of economic growth and industrial leadership. As part of

---

[1] A project to foster studies on two neglected diseases, leishmaniasis and Chagas, in collaboration with my Latin American academic partners.

[2] As defined by Rozenkopf, Sjatil and Stern (2019), a mission – a concrete, ambitious goal – has the power to unite different stakeholders to collaborate at scale and provide a bold and inspirational space to answer innovation challenges.

this framework, the Innovative Medicine Initiative, a public–private partnership between the EU and the pharmaceutical industry, supported several projects, including measures to combat infectious diseases such as Ebola (Laverty & Meulien, 2019). Investments included developing and testing a new vaccine against Ebola and community engagement to educate and assist in vaccine uptake in affected areas.

Considering the strength of the evidence, previous studies point to different directions in relation to the effectiveness of such public–private partnerships. In the case of PDPs and mission-driven innovation, despite the enormous literature on the management of these programmes, we still need a better understanding of how to implement them effectively (Uyarra et al., 2020). When it comes to defining the mission and using strategic purchasing in the public sector, we cannot ignore that asymmetries in information, market power, political power and financial power can hinder the effective implementation of these public–private partnerships (Corporate Europe Observatory, 2020; Greer, Klasa & van Ginneken, 2020). Particularly in the health sector, with the introduction of new medical treatments, policymakers and regulators must decide on medicines whose effectiveness is low or even controversial, as in the case of Aducanumab (Salinas, 2021). Scholars have proposed different scenarios in which public purchasing can promote economic development and structural change (Uyarra et al., 2020) and methodologies as to remedy this limitation (Héder, 2017).

Although stimulating drug production in LMICs could bring potential cost savings, as some locally produced pharmaceuticals are less expensive than their imported versions, there is no consensus about this dilemma (Chaves et al., 2015; Kaplan, 2011). The tension between two objectives cannot be ignored: access to medicines depends not just on procuring at the lowest price, but also on having a stable supply of vaccine and drugs (Shadlen & Fonseca, 2013). Kaplan (2011) found some evidence that investments in local pharmaceutical production increased the innovative capacity of local firms, particularly in Southeast Asian countries, and other modest innovation experiences in sub-Saharan Africa. In the case of antiretroviral drug production, clearly the local production of medicines increased the export capacity of India and South Africa, but there was little evidence that local production increased the quality standards for the product or the reliability of supply in LMICs.

Finally, considering the alliance between these two realms – health care and industry – we cannot ignore the challenges of coordination.

Brazil is a successful case in which government commitments in health, which often translate into public procurement for essential health supplies, revealed weaknesses and deficiencies in manufacturing of pharmaceutical products and incentivized industrial development in sectors where demand is strong (Flynn, 2014; Nunn, 2008; Shadlen & Fonseca, 2013). However, the case of India is illustrative as the country is known worldwide for its impressive drug industry, which has contributed to increasing access to medicines in several LMICs but has so far failed to provide essential medicines regularly to its own people (Chaudhuri, 2007). China, a giant producer of active pharmaceutical ingredients, also failed to provide satisfactory pharmaceutical care in its national health system but has recently begun applying strategies to remedy this situation (Abbott, 2017). During the COVID-19 pandemic, despite the vaccine development capacity of China, India and Russia, all three struggled to achieve high immunization rates quickly (Safi, Merz & Davidson, 2021). All these examples suggest we still need to better understand which channels, governance arrangements, and mechanisms can promote effective coordination between health care and industrial capabilities. Such challenges are not easy to overcome and will require continuous debates in forums such as the WLPF.

Co-benefits between SDG3 and SDG9 should produce spillover effects on other SDGs as well. For instance, the policies discussed so far have clear implications for SDG17 (global partnership for sustainable development), which promotes public–private partnerships, multilateral cooperation, and science, technology and innovation capacity-building mechanisms. Over the past two decades, vaccine R&D has been transformed by public–private partnerships such as DNDi and GAVI (a global partnership that provides vaccines to low-income countries), combining the strengths of both sides to develop, finance and deliver affordable vaccines to children in LMIC.

Fig. 9.1 depicts some of the causal pathways between health systems and industrial, innovation and infrastructure actions. Specifically, it illustrates these pathways in the initiative to stimulate local production of pharmaceuticals, diagnostics and vaccines in LMICs. Between the two extremes – health and industrial goals – there are several intersectoral actions ("enabling ecosystems"), such as strengthening the regulatory capacity that is necessary to assess good manufacturing practices. There is a need to promote partnerships such as South–South cooperation or technology transfer, continuous training of human resources, and

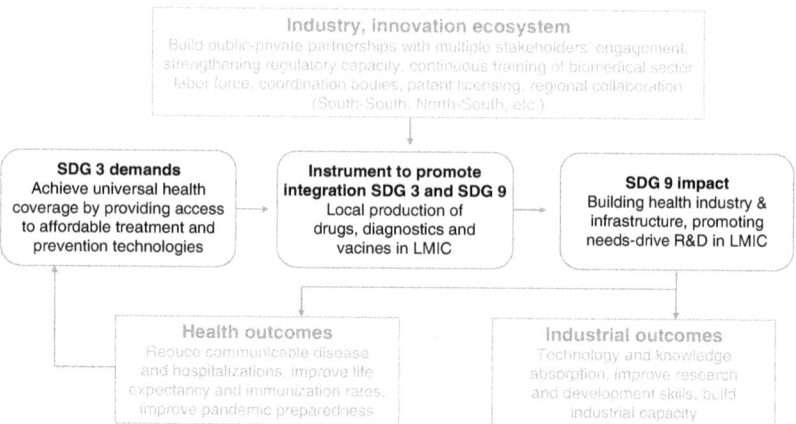

Fig. 9.1 Mapping causal pathways between health programmes and co-benefits

absorption of new knowledge and technology for drug and vaccine production. Achieving SDG9 goals will produce industrial outcomes such as technology absorption, but also health benefits such as the reduction of communicable disease transmission because of increased access to vaccines (as in the case of hepatitis B), improvement of pandemic preparedness, and eventually improvement of population health outcomes (for example, reduced hospitalizations and increased life expectancy and immunization rates).

9.4 Case study 1: HPV vaccine technology transfer in Brazil

This section discusses Brazil's technology transfer strategy for the HPV vaccine. HPV is one of the most common sexually transmitted infections, and a small percentage of infections, depending on the viral type, can progress to cervical cancer. Cervical cancer is the fourth most common cancer in women, with 85% of new cases occurring in LMIC, and 87% of deaths from cervical cancer occurring in less-developed regions (Ferlay et al., 2015). Brazil introduced HPV vaccination into the National Immunization Programme (PNI) in 2014, after the approval of the National Commission of Technology Incorporation (Conitec) (Domingues, Maranhão & Soares Pinto, 2015). In 2012, the Ministry of Health encouraged the transfer of HPV vaccine technology from Merck Sharp & Dohme (MSD) to a local, state-owned laboratory, the

Butantan Institute, as a way of maintaining a stable, affordable supply of vaccines (Baker et al., 2015).[3] Promoting access to HPV vaccination and technology transfer relates directly to SDG3.3 (fight communicable disease), 3.8 (achieve universal health care coverage), and 3b (support research, development and universal access to affordable vaccines). It also creates relevant co-benefits relating to SDG9 (industry, innovation and infrastructure) and SDG5 (gender equality).

The transfer of HPV vaccine technology is part of Brazil's strategy to use the purchasing power of the health system to stimulate transfer of knowledge and technology around drug and vaccine production to local firms (public and private) (Varrichio, 2017). In 2012, the Ministry of Health opened a call for partners interested in transferring HPV vaccine technology to a public laboratory. Two consortia submitted a proposal: GlaxoSmithKlein and Biomanguinhos, with a bivalent (protects against two virus types) HPV vaccine, and MSD and Butantan, with a quadrivalent (against four virus types) HPV vaccine. After deliberation by the Management Commission, which included representatives of the National Health Surveillance Agency as well as the Ministries of Health, of Industry and Trade, and of Science and Technology, the Ministry of Health approved the MSD/Butantan consortium, arguing that a quadrivalent vaccine was a better technology. In addition, the agreement with Butantan included access to the nonavalent (against nine types) portfolio which was then under research (Gadelha, 2018). A total of US$452.5 million would be invested in purchasing the vaccine over a five-year period, starting in 2014, while the technology was being transferred (Marchesini, 2013).

The technology transfer arrangement proceeded in reverse, from the final to the early stages of the production process. Between 2014 and 2016, Butantan was responsible for importing vaccines from MSD and distributing them to the Ministry of Health. In 2016, Butantan proceeded to fill and finish the product, certify quality control, and package the medicine for distribution (Albuquerque, 2016). Although the Ministry of Health and the government of São Paulo agreed to invest R$300 million (US$54.4 million) to build a new factory for Butantan, which would allow the full transfer of the HPV technology (Marchesini, 2013), the project is yet to be finished.

---

[3] Vaccine efficacy can be accessed here: https://www.merckvaccines.com/gardasil9/efficacy/#Demo27to45 (accessed 15 November 2021).

The governance structure of the HPV agreement specified Ministry of Health involvement primarily in coordination, monitoring and evaluation of the partnership, guiding technology transfer protocols, and financing. The CGU (Office of the Comptroller General) and the TCU (Federal Court of Accounts) audit the PDP contracts (including the HPV vaccine technology transfer) and set parameters for them (Table 9.1). However, the partnership stalled owing to low access to the capital needed to build the new factory (the final step to conclude knowledge transfer). It illustrates, therefore, the challenges of securing governments' long-term commitment to local drug production and the crucial relevance of access to credit for the sustainability of technology transfer projects.

The HPV vaccine technology transfer produced important co-benefits in terms of industry, innovation and infrastructure. These benefits correspond particularly to SDG Targets 9.2 (promote inclusive and sustainable industrialization) and 9.5 (enhance research and upgrade

Table 9.1 *Governance actions and intersectoral structures of the HPV vaccine technology transfer*

Tools			Governance actions								
			Goals and targets	Evidence support	Policy guidance	Implementation and management	Coordination	Advocacy	Monitoring and evaluation	Financial support	Legal mandate
Tools	Plan	Plan (agreement)	x			x	x		X	X	x
	Indicators and targets	Indicators									
		Targets									
	Budgeting	Pooled budget									
		Shared objectives	x		x			x	x		
		Coordinated budgeting	x			x				x	x

Table 9.1 *(Cont.)*

			Governance actions							
Tools	**Organization**	Ministry of Health	x		x	x		x	x	x
		CONITEC		x						
		Ministerial linkages (Industry and Trade, Science and Technology, ANVISA)						x		
		Butantan (State-owned laboratory)		x						
		Regional government (Sao Paulo)					x			
		MSD		x						
	Accountability	Transparent data	x							
		Regular reporting	x					x		
		Independent agency/ evaluators: TCU and CGU	x	x	x					x
		Support for civil society								
		Legal rights								

industrial technologies). According to a representative of the Ministry of Health who participated in the HPV agreement, the technology transfer would not only allow sustainable, affordable access to the HPV vaccine, but would also modernize Butantan's technological capacity, which was then dedicated to an outdated product portfolio (Gadelha, 2018). In terms of industrial and innovation goals, the technology transfer of the HPV vaccine brought important gains to Butantan. First, it allowed Butantan to make use of the Virus-like Particle (VLP) vaccine platform (Kallil, 2018). In possession of technology that uses VLPs – molecules that mimic viruses but are not infectious – Butantan would be able to conduct research in new directions. Noteworthily, after almost ten years of agreement, the factory was not built, causing delays to Butantan's full assimilation of the technology. Second, in terms of quality and process control, Butantan has undergone notable advancement in its infrastructure as part of this agreement, an improvement reflected in the manufacturing of other products as well. For instance, it has enhanced quality control processes in production of the influenza vaccine (Rocca, 2018). For MSD, besides gaining access to the Brazilian market, the partnership was important in that it certified an additional outsource supply, which is significant considering that production is a major bottleneck in the vaccine supply chain (Lesser, 2014).

Besides the co-benefits in industry and innovation, the technology transfer of the HPV vaccine and vaccination also produced spillover effects on gender equality, particularly in ensuring access to sexual and reproductive health (SDG Target 5.6) (Portnoy et al., 2020). Therefore, as younger females have higher rates of vaccination in Brazil (Wendland et al., 2021), it can evidence their access to sexual and reproductive health care. The technology transfer of the HPV vaccine was also an important instrument to stimulate public–private partnerships in the health sector (SDG Target 17.17, encourage effective public–private partnerships).

The HPV vaccine technology transfer took place in a context of expansion of health industry policies in Brazil (Shadlen & Fonseca, 2013). Although public laboratories such as Butantan and Biomanguinhos had engaged in technology transfer of vaccines in the past, in 2011 the Ministry of Health began an ambitious project, known as PDP, to foster technological development of local pharmaceutical companies. The legal architecture and protocols of PDPs paved the way for the transfer of HPV vaccine technology. Given the strategic relevance of the HPV vaccine to the public health system and its technological gains to Brazil and Butantan, the political importance of this project can be defined as high. The political conflict, in contrast, is defined as low, as there was collaboration between the government of São Paulo and the Ministry of Health, as well as a voluntary patent licence awarded to Butantan. The latter is usually a key source of contention in the pharmaceutical sector. By promoting an agreement with Butantan, MSD has gained market access to Brazil's public health system and certified a new outsource supplier (Table 9.2).

Table 9.2 *Political importance and conflict: the context of policymaking and implementation of HPV technology transfer*

		Conflict	
		Low	High
Political	High	x	
importance	Low		

9.5 Case study 2: the Mozambican Pharmaceutical Ltd: a South–South cooperation project

In 2003, the governments of Brazil (henceforth GoB) and Mozambique (GoM) signed a South–South cooperation (SSC) agreement for the installation of the *Sociedade Moçambicana de Medicamentos* (SMM, or Mozambican Pharmaceutical Ltd), a pharmaceutical laboratory for the production of antiretroviral (ARV) and other medications. Based on Brazil's successful domestic production of ARV generics to fight the HIV/AIDS epidemics, the SMM would also help foster Mozambique's – and sub-Saharan Africa's – first state-owned pharmaceutical industry. Local production of medicine through capacity-building courses and technology transfer from Brazil is directly related to – and could potentially produce – the SDG Targets 3.3 (fight communicable disease), 3.8 (increase access to quality and affordable essential medicines), 3b (support the research and development of vaccines and medicines), and 3c (increase health financing and the recruitment, development, training and retention of the health workforce in developing countries). It could also produce co-benefits related to SDG9 (promotion of industrialization, innovation and infrastructure) and SDG17 (partnerships for the goal), particularly 17.6 (enhance SSC for access to science, technology and innovation, and enhance knowledge sharing on mutually agreed terms) and 17.9 (through SSC, enhance international support for implementing effective and targeted capacity-building in developing countries). The implementation of the SMM unfolded in a low-income setting highly dependent on Indian generics. As such, this study may help illustrate how to increase access to medicines through domestic production in similar contexts in sub-Saharan Africa.

It can be argued that the implementation of the SMM went through three phases (Achcar, 2022). The initial phase was characterized by a common understanding among stakeholders of the importance of the factory in public health policies, particularly regarding the fight against HIV/AIDS, and the role of each institution in the governance of the SMM. On Brazil's side, the elaboration and implementation were carried out within the organizational structure of Brazil's SSC. The project was formally coordinated by the Brazilian Cooperation Agency (ABC) under the Ministry of Foreign Affairs (MRE), with Fiocruz[4] as the implementing agency, specifically the Institute of Drug Technology (Farmanguinhos)[5] (Table 9.3). Because ABC's capacity was low and coordination was still weak, the "true centre of gravity of Brazilian health cooperation" was the Ministry of Health, particularly Fiocruz (Abdenur & Folly, 2015).

In Mozambique, the factory belongs to a public business institution called the Institute for the Management of State Holdings (Portuguese acronym, IGEPE), and the sectorial tutelage is exercised by Mozambique's MoH (also called MISAU) (Table 9.3). IGEPE was created in 2001 to restructure state-owned enterprises and determine the sectors in which state ownership was considered necessary (Balbuena, 2014). Despite being the formal owner and financial tutor of the factory since 2009, it was not until the change in the Ministers of Health in 2010 (second phase) that IGEPE started playing a key role in the management of the factory (Achcar, 2022). Although not openly contested, this was a point of disagreement between the two governments. According to Fiocruz's health experts, the governance of the SMM should ideally model that of Brazil and Farmanguinhos. In other words, the SMM should belong to Mozambique's MoH and as such should be 100% state-owned (Achcar, 2022).

Although in the first phase both governments agreed that the SMM should be 100% state-owned, in the second phase the GoM desired to privatize it. Without yielding financial results, the longest and most expensive Brazilian SSC project in health needed public investment that the GoM claimed not to have. The Brazilian mining giant Vale stepped in and financed the infrastructure (Russo & Oliveira, 2016). Another obstacle to the implementation of the factory was Brazil's delay in approving the funds necessary to buy the equipment for the factory. Brazil did not possess a legal framework for SSC, which made the

[4] Fiocruz is the Oswaldo Cruz Foundation, Brazil's largest public health institute.
[5] Farmanguinhos is currently the largest official pharmaceutical laboratory linked to the Ministry of Health.

Table 9.3 *Governance actions and intersectoral structures of SMM South-South collaboration*

Tools			Governance actions								
			Goals and targets	Evidence support	Policy guidance	Implementation and management	Coordination	Advocacy	Monitoring and evaluation	Financial support	Legal mandate
	Plan	Plan	x			x	x		x		x
	Indicators and targets	Indicators									
		Targets									
	Budgeting	Pooled budget									
		Shared objectives									
		Coordinated budgeting									
	Organization	In Brazil									
		Ministry of Foreign Affairs (MRE)	x		x		x				
		Brazilian Cooperation Agency (ABC)	x		x		x		x[6]		
		Ministry of Health (MoH)			x	x					
		Fiocruz/ Farmanguinhos	x			x	x				
		Anvisa	x		x	x					x
		Private Sector (Vale)								x	
		National Congress								x[7]	x

[6] Brazilian SSC is criticized for the absence of a systematic MandE. It would be the ABC's responsibility to provide MandE, with the MoH and Fiocruz also exercising some monitoring along the way.

[7] Approval of financial support for purchasing equipment.

Table 9.3 (*Cont.*)

			Governance actions					
			In Mozambique					
Tools	Accountability	Ministry of Health (MISAU)	x	x	x	x		x[8]
		Regulatory Agency (DNF)		x	x			x
		IGEPE	x			x		
		Mozambique Stock Exchange (private capital)					x	
		Transparent data	x					
		Regular reporting	x					
		Independent agency/ evaluators: TCU and CGU[9] (In Brazil)	x	x	x			x
		Support for civil society						
		Legal rights						

allocation of resources into projects very difficult. It took the National Congress 20 months to approve the funds.

When the desire to privatize the SMM became clearer to Brazil, there was intense mobilization from the MRE, the MoH and, especially, Fiocruz to convince the GoM of the strategic importance of the factory not only to the health system but also to the development of a nascent national industry (Achcar, 2022), thus closely connecting it to SDG9.

---

[8] The financial support from MISAU would come from public purchases of drugs.
[9] Both TCU (Federal Court of Accounts) and CGU (Office of the Comptroller General) provide internal oversight of agencies such as Fiocruz, including its SSC initiatives. The TCU audits the accounts related to SSC – for example, the funds approved by the National Congress for equipment for the SMM.

It was argued that this would promote spillover effects on different sectors of the economy owing to high technology development and transfer and the creation of high-quality employment. The argument was based on Brazil's – particularly Fiocruz's – view that integrating health policy objectives and industrial policies was crucial (Fonseca, 2018). Furthermore, throughout the project the importance of the SSC for the promotion of self-sustainability was always emphasized, reinforcing arguments related to SDG17.

Another important event reinforced the importance of today's SDG9. HIV underwent mutations and Brazil no longer had the technology to produce the most modern ARV drug. The decision, agreed upon by both sides, was to transfer the technology required for the production of essential medicines in primary health care only. This, according to Fiocruz and the MoH, was not a negative decision. Producing essential medicines would spearhead the production of other technologies (Achcar, 2022).

The third and final phase in the implementation of the SMM was characterized by a compromise between the two governments over the fate of the SMM. Rather than being 100% state-owned, the governments reached a common decision whereby 35% of the SMM's shares were to be listed in the country's stock exchange to raise capital while preserving majority state ownership. A few recent initiatives in 2020 seemed to strengthen the SMM's role in enhancing a local pharmaceutical industry, namely 1) negotiations for public–private partnerships with foreign laboratories, 2) the implementation of a health regulatory agency with the support of Brazil's health regulatory agency, Anvisa, and 3) the successful application for membership of the Southern African Generic Medicines Association (SAGMA). While the political significance of the SMM was high for Brazil's SSC foreign policy strategy, it can be classified as moderate for Mozambique. The political conflict between the two countries can be classified as moderate to low, as both governments reached an agreement in the end (Table 9.4).

9.6 Conclusion

The editors define co-benefits as the intended positive side-effects of a policy from subsidiary benefits, i.e., unintended positive side-effects. In other words, co-benefits are secondary benefits, collateral benefits or associated benefits. In this chapter, we argued that adopting initiatives

Table 9.4 *Political importance and conflict: the context of policymaking and implementation of the SMM*

Brazil		Conflict	
		Low	Medium
Political importance	High		x
	Low		

Mozambique		Conflict	
		Low	Medium
Political importance	High		
	Medium		x
	Low		

for technology transfer and local production of vaccines and drugs can lead to a stable supply of pharmaceuticals, which, in turn, can generate capability gains for the pharmaceutical sectors. By fostering local production, countries will be encouraged to strengthen their regulatory systems, which is crucial to manufacturing practices, and ensure quality control. It will also be an opportunity to train and develop human resources, develop new skills, and promote local industrial development. Although the pathways to achieve co-benefits are relatively straightforward, the practice of transferring knowledge and gaining pharmaceutical manufacturing capabilities is more complex.

For decades, the WHO has incentivized LMICs to invest in needs-driven R&D and local drug production. The SDG Target 3b reflects the global consensus on the relevance of fostering drug manufacturing capabilities in LMICs. Despite the WHO reports, guidelines and studies, LMICs still struggle to fully accomplish these goals.

The cases of the HPV vaccine and the SMM illustrate that these projects can suffer from delays and shortages of funding, which can negatively affect the full assimilation of technology and industrial development. Both projects have produced relevant intermediate benefits, and interviewees have demonstrated a great appreciation for technology and manufacturing gains. Therefore, although technology transfer is valuable, it is easier said than done (Fonseca, Shadlen & Bastos, 2021; O'Sullivan, Rutten & Schatz, 2020).

With the renewed interest in local drug production in LMICs as a means of scaling up COVID-19 vaccine production (Fonseca, Shadlen

& Achcar, 2023; O'Sullivan, Rutten & Schatz, 2020; WHO, 2021b) and the popularity of mission-driven innovation policies (fostered mainly by the European Union) (European Commission, 2015; European Union, 2019), we will need to reflect on effective ways to implement these initiatives on the ground. The first step is to look back at the past and avoid similar mistakes. The GSPA-PHI assessment report recognized the lack of impact in its implementation and proposed focused actions (WHO, 2018). Therefore, initiatives such as the WHO's World Local Production Forum – a global platform to foster discussions about local production of pharmaceuticals, vaccines and other health products – must produce clear goals and targets.

Another vital aspect is the acknowledgement that the political economy is critical, especially in a highly politicized environment such as the biomedical sector. As the case study from Brazil shows, private–public collaboration can result in mutual benefits.

The first step of technology transfer is defining what knowledge will be transferred and why. This knowledge is typically framed as a strategic product that is crucial in life-saving terms and essential for health security. Yet, as we learned from other experiences, the concept of "strategic" cannot be taken for granted given the asymmetries in the pharmaceutical sector (Greer, Klasa & van Ginnekin, 2020). The same is true for drug regulatory capacity, which is still incipient in many countries in the Global South (Khadem Broojerdi et al., 2020). Without robust health and manufacturing surveillance, any attempt to produce drugs and vaccines in LMICs will be insufficient.

Therefore, technology transfer and local production require good governance practices, such as coordination among government departments, conducive regulatory policies, complementary supply-side measures, clearly articulated policy objectives, and careful evaluation, which are framed as "enabling ecosystems". Perhaps no other public policy requires the political ability to build coalitions with different stakeholders in such complex value chains while also building new governance capabilities in sensitive areas (for example, public budgets and patents). Doing so can be even more challenging in the context of LMICs. Not all countries have such ecosystems, and some countries only possess an informal network of players engaged in production, research and particular aspects of innovation. Technology and knowledge transfer can help foster these ecosystems and achieve the SDG9 targets.

References

Abbott F (2017). China policies to promote local production of pharmaceutical products and protect public health. Geneva: World Health Organization, 2–17.

Abdenur AE, Folly M (2015). The new development bank and the institutionalization of the BRICS. BRICS-Studies and Documents, 77–111.

Achcar HM (2022). South-South Cooperation and the re-politicization of development in health. World Dev, 149:105679. (https://doi.org/10.1016/j.worlddev.2021.105679)

Albuquerque F (2016, 15 June). Butantan apresenta transferência de tecnologia para produzir vacina contra HPV [Butantan presents technology transfer to produce HPV vaccine]. Agencia Brasil.

Baker M, Figueroa-Downing D, Chiang E et al. (2015). Paving pathways: Brazil's implementation of a national human papillomavirus immunization campaign. *Rev Panam Salud Publica*, 36(2):163–166.

Balbuena SS (2014). State-owned enterprises in Southern Africa: a stocktaking of reforms and challenges.

Chaudhuri S (2007). The Gap Between Successful Innovation and Access to Its Benefits: Indian Pharmaceuticals. Eur J Dev Res, 19(1):49–65.

Chaves C, Hasenclever L, Serpa C et al. (2015). Estratégias de redução de preços de medicamentos para aids em situação de monopólio no Brasil [Strategies to reduce prices of AIDS drugs in a monopoly situation in Brazil]. Rev Saude Publica, 49(86):1–11.

Corporate Europe Observatory (2020). More private than public: the ways Big Pharma dominates the Innovative Medicines Initiative. (https://corporateeurope.org/sites/default/files/2020-05/IMI-report-final_0.pdf)

Directorate-General for Research and Innovation (2003). Raising EU R&D Intensity: Improving the Effectiveness of the Mix of Public Support Mechanisms for Private Sector Research and Development. Brussels: European Commission.

Domingues C, Maranhão A, Soares Pinto M (2015). The introduction of HPV vaccines in Brazil: Advances and challenges. DST – J bras Doenças Sexualmente Transmissíveis, 27(34):67–72.

Drugs for Neglected Diseases initiative (2019). 15 Years of needs-driven innovation for access. (https://dndi.org/publications/2019/15-years-of-needs-driveninnovation-for-access/)

European Commission (2015). Press Release: European public-private partnerships delivering first socio-economic impacts. Brussels: European Commission.

European Union (2019). Innovation Procurement: The power of the public purse. Brussels: European Union.

Ferlay J, Soerjomataram I, Dikshit R et al. (2015). Cancer incidence and mortality worldwide: Sources, methods and major patterns in GLOBOCAN 2012. Int J Cancer, 136(5):E359–E386. (doi: https://doi.org/10.1002/ijc.29210)

Flynn M (2014). Pharmaceutical autonomy and public health in Latin America: State, society and industry in Brazil's AIDS Program. London: Routledge.

Flynn M (2015). Pharmaceutical autonomy and public health in Latin America: State, society and industry in Brazil's AIDS Program. New York: Routledge.

Fonseca EM, Shadlen KC, Achcar HdM (2023). Vaccine technology transfer in a global health crisis: Actors, capabilities, and institutions. Res Policy, 52(4):104739. (doi: https://doi.org/10.1016/j.respol.2023.104739)

Fonseca EM, Shadlen KC, Bastos FI (2021). The politics of COVID-19 vaccination in middle-income countries: Lessons from Brazil. Soc Sci Med, 281:114093. (doi: https://doi.org/10.1016/j.socscimed.2021.114093)

Gadelha CAG (2003). O complexo industrial da saúde e a necessidade de um enfoque dinâmico na economia da saúde. *Ciência & saúde coletiva*, 8:521–535.

Gadelha C (2018). Interview with Elize Massard da Fonseca on 7 March, Rio de Janeiro.

Greer S, Klasa K, van Ginneken E (2020). Power and Purchasing: Why Strategic Purchasing Fails. Milbank Q, 98(3):975–1020. (doi: https://doi.org/10.1111/1468-0009.12471)

Héder M (2017). From NASA to EU: the evolution of the TRL scale in Public Sector Innovation. Innov J, 22:1–13.insights/europe/how-purpose-led-missions-can-help-europe-innovate-at-scale)

Kallil J (2018). Interview with Elize Massard da Fonseca on 13 March, Sao Paulo.

Kaplan W (2011). Local production and access to medicines in low- and middle-income countries: a literature review and critical analysis. Geneva: World Health Organization.

Khadem Broojerdi A, Baran Sillo H, Ostad Ali Dehaghi R et al. (2020). The World Health Organization Global Benchmarking Tool: an Instrument to Strengthen Medical Products Regulation and Promote Universal Health Coverage. Front Med, 7(457).

Kok W (2004). Facing the Challenge. The Lisbon Strategy for Growth and Employment. Report from a High Level Group. Luxembourg: Office for Official Publications of the European Communities.

Kynčlová P, Upadhyaya S, Nice T (2020). Composite index as a measure on achieving Sustainable Development Goal 9 (SDG-9) industry-related targets: The SDG-9 index. Appl Energy, 265:114755. (doi: https://doi.org/10.1016/j.apenergy.2020.114755)

Laverty H, Meulien P (2019). The Innovative Medicines Initiative – 10 Years of Public-Private Collaboration. Front Med, 6:275. (doi: 10.3389/fmed.2019.00275).

Lesser G (2014). Interview with Elize Massard da Fonseca on 14 October, Sao Paulo.

Mackintosh M, Banda G, Tibandebage P et al. (eds). (2016). Making medicines in Africa: The Political Economy of Industrializing for Local Health. New York: Palgrave Macmillan.

Marchesini L (2013, 1 July). Governo destina R$ 1 bi para vacina contra HPV [Government allocates R$1 billion for HPV vaccine]. Valor Economico.

Natera J, Tomassini C, Vera-Cruz A (2019). Policy analysis and knowledge application for building a healthy health innovation system in developing countries. Innov Dev, 9(2):159–168.

Nunn A (2008). The politics and history of AIDS treatment in Brazil. New York: Springer.

Nunn A, Fonseca E, Gruskin S (2009). Changing Global Essential Medicines Norms to Improve Access to AIDS Treatment: Lessons from Brazil. Glob Public Health, 4(2):117.

O'Sullivan C, Rutten P, Schatz C (2020). Why tech transfer may be critical to beating COVID-19. (https://www.mckinsey.com/industries/pharmaceuticals-and-medical-products/ourinsights/why-tech-transfer-may-be-critical-to-beating-covid-19)

Portnoy A, Clark S, Ozawa S et al. (2020). The impact of vaccination on gender equity: conceptual framework and human papillomavirus (HPV) vaccine case study. Int J Equity Health, 19(1):10. (doi:10.1186/s12939-019-1090-3)

Proksch D, Busch-Casler J, Haberstroh M et al. (2019). National health innovation systems: Clustering the OECD countries by innovative output in healthcare using a multi indicator approach. Res Policy, 48:169–179.

Rocca T (2018). Interview with Elize Massard da Fonseca on 13 August, Sao Paulo.

Rozenkopf I, Sjatil P, Stern S (2019). How purpose-led missions can help Europe innovate at scale. (https://www.mckinsey.com/featured-insights/europe/how-purpose-led-missions-can-help-europe-innovate-at-scale)

Russo G, Banda G (2015). Re-Thinking Pharmaceutical Production in Africa; Insights from the Analysis of the Local Manufacturing Dynamics in Mozambique and Zimbabwe. Stud Comp Int Dev, 50(2):258–281.

Russo G, de Oliveira L (2016). South-South collaboration in pharmaceuticals: Manufacturing anti-retroviral medicines in Mozambique. *Making Medicines in Africa: The Political Economy of Industrializing for Local Health*, 85–102.

Safi M, Merz T, Davidson H (2021, 26 March). Why home-produced Covid vaccine hasn't helped India, Russia and China rollouts. *The Guardian*.

(https://www.theguardian.com/world/2021/mar/17/why-covid-vaccine-home-producedindia-russia-china-slow-start)

Salinas R (2021). Aducanumab for Alzheimer's disease: expediting approval and delaying science. BMJ Evid Based Med, 26(5):214. doi:10.1136/bmjebm-2021-111765.

Santiago F (2020). Turning health challenges into industrialization opportunities for developing countries. (https://iap.unido.org/articles/turning-health-challengesindustrialization-opportunities-developing-countries)

Shadlen K, Fonseca E (2013). Health Policy as Industrial Policy: Brazil in Comparative Perspective. Polit Soc, 41(4):560–586.

United Nations Economic and Social Council (2016). Progress towards the Sustainable Development Goals: Report of the Secretary-General. (https://www.un.org/ga/search/view_doc.asp?symbol=E/2016/75&Lang=E)

Uyarra E, Zabala-Iturriagagoitia J, Flanagan K et al. (2020). Public procurement, innovation and industrial policy: Rationales, roles, capabilities and implementation. Res Policy, 49(1):103844.

Varrichio P (2017). As parcerias para o desenvolvimento produtivo da saúde [Partnerships for the productive development of health]. In: Rauen A (ed.) Políticas de inovação pelo lado da demanda no Brasil. Brasília: IPEA.

Wendland EM, Kops NL, Bessel M et al. (2021). Effectiveness of a universal vaccination program with an HPV quadrivalent vaccine in young Brazilian women. Vaccine, 39(13):1840–1845. (doi: https://doi.org/10.1016/j.vaccine.2021.02.040)

WHO (2011). Local production for access to medical products: developing a framework to improve public health. Geneva: World Health Organization.

WHO (2018). Overall programme review of the global strategy and plan of action on public health, innovation and intellectual property. Report of the review panel. (https://apps.who.int/iris/handle/10665/273827)

WHO (2021a). At Local Production Forum, WHO and partners highlight key steps to improve access to health technologies [Press release]. (https://www.who.int/news/item/25-06-2021-at-local-production-forum-who-andpartners-highlight-key-steps-to-improve-access-to-health-technologies)

WHO (2021b). World Local Production Forum: Enhancing access to medicines and other health technologies: Brochure for Speakers. Geneva: World Health Organization.

World Health Assembly (2008). Global strategy and plan of action on public health, innovation and intellectual property. Geneva: World Health Organization.

10 | SDG10, reduced inequalities: the effect of health policy on inequalities: evidence from South Africa

OGUJIUBA KANAYO, OLAIDE OJONIYI

10.1 Introduction

South Africa remains racially and economically segregated, despite the end of apartheid in the early 1990s. The country is plagued by persistent social inequality, poverty, unemployment, a high disease burden, and inequitable health care service provision. The South African health system is currently engaged in the complex project of establishing universal health coverage, which ensures the system's ability to provide comprehensive care that is accessible, affordable and acceptable to patients and families while acknowledging the system's significant pressures. Nonetheless, inequalities in post-apartheid South Africa have been extensively analysed, yet not much has happened as to the effect of health policy on inequalities in the country. This chapter provides an overview of the effects of health policy on inequalities in South Africa, emphasizing how SDG3 (health for all) and SDG10 (reduce inequalities) can fight the long-term societal inequalities. It explains the inequalities in South Africa, the country's available health policies, and how this has affected the long-existing trend in the country. South Africa is one of the most unequal countries in the world. The country's Gini coefficient is high and the highest among countries with comparable characteristics. The 10% richest of the population spend 7.9 times more than the 40% at the base. The inequality started during the apartheid period when racial separation was legislated and was a strategic area of policy concentration for the first democratic government. Today, years after the end of apartheid, though there is a decline, the country still battles to fix the differences despite sustained positive economic growth. The issue persists with racial footprint. The divide is visible in social, economic and health areas. This chapter aims to demonstrate the capacity for social innovation in health concerning South Africa and to highlight some current innovations that respond to issues of health equity, such as accessibility, affordability and acceptability.

10.2 Background

Transformative change is required to reduce inequality. Greater efforts are required to eradicate extreme poverty and hunger, as well as increased investment in health, education, social protection and decent jobs, particularly for young people, migrants and refugees, and other vulnerable communities. Thus, the United Nations General Assembly in 2015 published the 17 Sustainable Development Goals intended to be achieved by the year 2030 by all countries. The goals are aimed at peace and prosperity for people and the planet, now and into the future. Importance is attached to how a reduction in deprivation goes together with plans to improve health, education, equality, the economy and the environment. The SDGs focus on development as well as on restoring the dignity of people. Before the United Nations' SDGs, South Africa adopted the National Development Plan (NDP): Vision 2030 in 2012. The NDP closely lines up with the SDGs. It focuses on minimizing inequality, growing an all-encompassing economy, and eradicating poverty by 2030. The goals are incorporated into government planning systems and processes at the national, provincial and local levels. SDG10 aims to reduce inequality within and between countries. It advocates for the reduction of income inequalities, as well as inequalities based on age, gender, disability, race, ethnicity, origin, religion or economic status. SDG10 to reduce inequality is also one of the priorities of the NDP. This is especially relevant to South Africa. Growing inequality impedes long-term development, slows economic growth, and undermines social cohesion within societies. There is no international agreement that reducing inequality is critical to ending poverty by 2030.

The non-White population has consistently been in the lowest income and wealth strata. Households in this group rely more on social grants, whereas those at the top rely on labour-market income, which is heavily racialized and gender-biased. The South African labour market contributes significantly to overall income inequality. Aside from having dire employment outcomes, Black Africans earn the lowest wages. Nearly half of the Black population lives below the poverty line, compared to less than 1% of the White population. Recently, it was reported that between

2009 and 2015 there was a consistent increase in the average number of assets owned by the Black population. However, asset inequality persists even within different quintiles of the Black population groups. Most households in South Africa do not have access to clean water, while at least 14% live in congested informal settlements. The apartheid system forced Black South Africans into informal housing settlements which were cut off from infrastructure and overcrowded. Since the emergence of democratic rule, the government has funded millions of new homes for Black South Africans but these houses were developed within the settlements, sustaining the geographical segregation created during apartheid (Fogel, 2019). These settlements have little access to public services and utilities. Nonetheless, a South African child's educational experience is still a function of place of birth, socioeconomic status and skin colour. The COVID-19 pandemic further exposed this as students from poor communities were cut off from education during the lockdown as a result of inadequate internet connection (Mohamed, 2021). The educational system is faced with clear inequalities and lingering underperformance. Schools are plagued with collapsing infrastructure, congested classrooms and poor educational outcomes. Students learn in schools with inadequate infrastructure and a lack of essential facilities. Some 75% of South Africa's schooling system consists of public schools situated in peri-urban and rural areas. These schools are attended mostly by poor Black children and are faced with overcrowding, poor resources and dysfunctionalities (Vally, 2020). Based on a government report in 2018, 19% of public schools use illegal pit latrines, 37 schools had no sanitation facilities; 86% had no laboratory; 77% had no library; 72% had no access to the internet and 42% had no sports facilities. As a result, education outcomes differ. Students in the topmost 200 schools get more distinctions in maths than students in all the preceding 6600 schools.

10.3   Causal pathways between health actions (policy) and SDG10 (reduce inequalities) co-benefits

Poverty, social and economic inequalities, and disparities in access to basic social services between population groups and provinces are common and symbolic in South Africa, and this helps to worsen inequalities in health (Ataguba, 2010; Coovadia et al., 2009). The South African government has employed a variety of strategies to combat the persistent levels of inequality that have troubled the nation. Higher social expenditure, targeted government transfers, and affirmative action to spread asset ownership and encourage entrepreneurship among the once-underprivileged have been the main strategies utilized to alleviate inequality (IMF, 2020). Inequalities in socioeconomic status in South Africa help to aggravate inequalities in health. This is because low socioeconomic status leads to deprivation (Ojoniyi et al., 2019). Studies on the burden of some disease conditions in the country have shown persistently that the poor suffer more from numerous diseases and violence than the rich. There is greater reporting of disease and disability among those in low socioeconomic classes compared to those in high socioeconomic classes (Ataguba, Akazili & McIntyre, 2011). There are specific benefits that can be gained from actions in the health system in reducing inequalities (SDG10). In this case, the benefits are twofold. Health policy in health can help in reducing inequalities in health outcomes, which in turn is an indication of the success of SDG3.

There is a link between SDG3 and SDG10, especially concerning universal health coverage. The health system influences the social determinants of health, enhancing health outcomes and tackling social inequalities (Gilson et al., 2007). To achieve this goal, the country aims to implement the National Health Insurance (NHI) and establish a unified health system. The NHI white paper prepared by the government of South Africa admits that good health is an essential state of humans' socioeconomic life and is a crucial precondition for poverty reduction, continued economic growth, and development. In a study conducted in the country, high socioeconomic status and perceived risk of HIV were associated with a decreased risk of infection (Mabaso et al., 2019). However, the link between universal health coverage and health inequality reduction is not so clear-cut, as it has been shown that higher socioeconomic groups use more services and have greater access to health care.

Also, the white paper recognizes that social factors contribute immensely towards improved health outcomes and long healthy life in the country. Poverty has been a principal factor promoting inequality in HIV prevalence among race groups created by historical and current unequal social and economic status in South Africa (Sia et al., 2014; Zembe et al., 2013). This requires a multisectoral approach to addressing social determinants of health. The NHI programme targets health promotion, prevention of disease, and empowering of communities. It

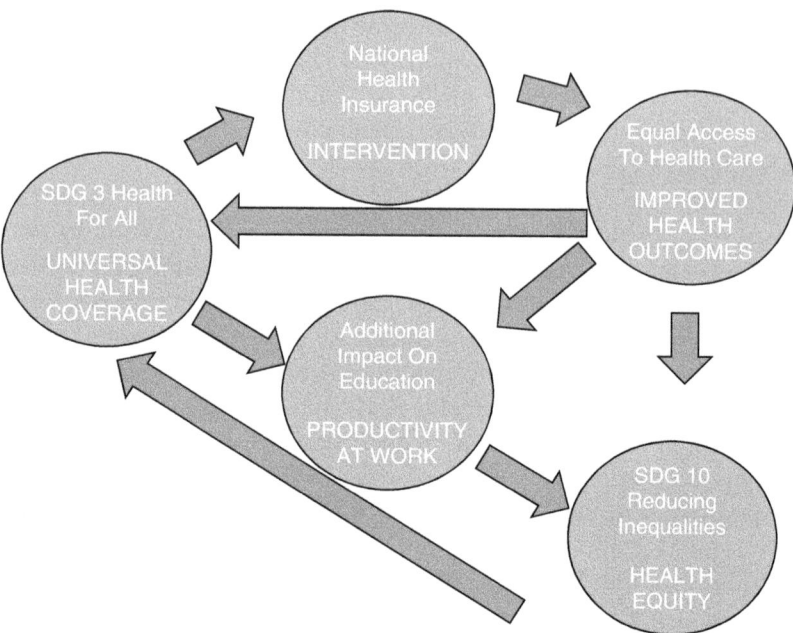

Fig. 10.1 Mapping proposed causal pathways between health policy and equality

intends to remove financial barriers to access to health care by transforming the financing of health services and extending population coverage.

Fig. 10.1 shows some of the pathways between SDG3 (health for all) and SDG10 (reducing inequalities). It starts with the NHI and continues with equal access to health care, which in turn contributes to SDG3, impacts education and productivity, and in turn impacts SDG10. Furthermore, there is a direct link from SDG10 to SDG3 in the medium to long term. Specifically, it depicts the pathways through which the NHI will help in reducing inequalities, particularly in health outcomes. The NHI is a health intervention aimed at reducing unequal access to quality health care, which will also result in better health outcomes, thereby achieving the goal of reducing inequality in health. Similarly, the health intervention will give room for equal access to quality health services irrespective of level of income, which will result in better health outcomes that will promote productivity at school and work with a resultant effect on educational and work outcomes. Improved educational and work outcomes will further reduce social inequalities.

Aside from the NHI scheme, the country has shown commitment to reducing inequality in the country. The first Voluntary National Review towards the realization of the SDGs shows the impact and programmes of the nation and multi-stakeholders' contributions to the achievement of the agenda. There has been an improvement in the living conditions of millions of South Africans: significant progress in education for children from poor households, with over 9 million children attending no-fee schools; more individuals now benefit from the social protection system (up to 17.5 million individuals in 2018); provision of clean water and electricity; over 4.5 million people benefit from the antiretroviral treatment programme which is the biggest in the world; increase in the representation of women in national parliament and legislature; and increasing actions to generate more employment (United Nations, 2019). However, high levels of inequalities, discrimination and violence against women remain.

10.4   Country case study

Since the end of apartheid 27 years ago, significant progress has been made in improving the lives of South Africans. The apartheid government's segregated population now has greater access to infrastructure and social amenities. However, the country is still battling apartheid-era racial segregation, inequalities and poverty. To reduce inequity and inequality, there is a need for equal access to public services. Poverty and employment status affect access to health care services and also have a great impact on nutrition and living conditions. South Africa has a well established economy and is classified as a middle-income country; since 2000, the average annual growth rate has been over 4.5%. Despite the economic growth, job creation and the wealth created are not evenly distributed. In South Africa, health care access for all is constitutionally protected, yet considerable inequities remain, largely due to distortions in resource allocation. Access barriers also include vast distances and high travel costs, especially in rural areas; high out-of-pocket payments for care; long queues; and disempowered patients (Harris et al., 2011). South Africa has four coexisting epidemics: poverty-related illnesses; maternal death and malnutrition; HIV/AIDS; and the growing burden of non-communicable diseases.

The origin of the dysfunctional health system and the collision of the epidemics of communicable and non-communicable diseases in South

Africa can be found in policies from various periods of the country's history, from colonial subjugation to apartheid dispossession to the post-apartheid period (Coovadia et al., 2009). The political, economic and land restriction policies during the apartheid era organized society by race, gender and age, which critically influenced the structure of family life and access to basic resources for health and health services. The unfair migration trajectory of rural male Black labourers to the towns was enforced by the economic situation at that time. Failure to provide proper housing for the migrant workers in urban areas led to the creation of overcrowded, unsanitary hostels and slums in the urban Black townships. Thus, the increased number of mine workers, and the repatriation of workers who were too ill to be productive, spread tuberculosis to the rural areas (Coovadia et al., 2009).

The SDGs at the global level and the NDP at the national and local levels give the country a platform from which to tackle its prevalent social problems. Both the SDGs and NDP target the year 2030. While the National department is responsible for policy formulation, the Department of Health, the caretaker of the South African health system, is a factor in the achievement of Priority 2 (education, skills and health) of the government's 2019–2024 Medium Term Strategic Framework, and the vision articulated in Chapter 10 of the NDP, such as reducing the burden of disease and strengthening the provision of health care to improve the lifespan of South Africans. Over the medium term, the Department of Health is expected to focus on carrying out the staged execution of NHI, investing in health infrastructure, preventing and treating communicable and non-communicable diseases, and financing tertiary hospital services. NHI is a system of health care funding in which all taxpayers or income earners make compulsory contributions, but the whole population is entitled to the benefits, including those who do not contribute. The introduction of the NHI scheme in South Africa is intended to push the health care system towards a socialized model – this is a state-supported service funded by taxation with little or no additional cost to the consumer. The purpose of the NHI is to cover the entire population with adequate health care at an affordable price. This system is not discriminatory. It is aimed at ensuring that everyone in South Africa has access to quality health services provided by both the public and private sectors irrespective of socioeconomic status. This system will reduce the disparity in health outcomes caused by inequality in socioeconomic status.

Table 10.1 *Governance actions and intersectoral structures of the National Health Insurance*

		Possible governance actions with these tools								
		Goals and targets	Evidence support	Policy guidance	Implementation and management	Coordination	Advocacy	Monitoring and evaluation	Financial support	Legal mandate
Plan	Plan	X						X		
Indicators and targets	Indicators	X						X		
	Targets	X						X		
Budgeting	Pooled budget								X	
	Shared objectives								X	
	Coordinated budgeting								X	
Organization	Ministerial linkages				X					X
	Specific ministers			X	X					X
	Organization			X	X					X
	Legislative committees	X		X	X					X
	Interdepartmental committees/units				X					X
	Departmental mergers				X					X
	Civic engagement				X		X		X	X
Accountability	Transparent data	X	X					X		
	Regular reporting	X	X					X		
	Independent agency/evaluators		X					X		
	Support for civil society									
	Legal rights									X

The NHI aims to increase access to high-quality health care for all South Africans, safeguard people financially from medical bills, and establish a public fund for all health services. To achieve the patient-centred, decentralized NHI that the government desires, a high level of organization and health service coordination is required. The government is to ensure that the constitution is met by finding all the resources available. The Health Professions Council of South Africa (HPCSA), on the other hand, is to ensure quality assurance, enforce professional codes of conduct and ethics, enhance human resources for health, and advocate for the proper regulation of private hospitals (National Health Insurance Bill, 2019).

The South African government started to implement the NHI in growing phases to secure public trust and improve public health services and infrastructures (Mkhize, 2019). It has been difficult to get public support for the scheme. The engagement of prominent leaders is required to get both public and political support for the implementation (Mkhize, 2019). The whole idea of the NHI is to gather public revenue to generate funds to eradicate inequality in access to health care between the private and public sectors (Onoka, Hanson & Hanefeld, 2015). The public has shown much concern about how much tax they will pay (National Health Insurance Bill, 2019). Hence, the government needs to show greater transparency and accountability on the matter.

The NHI programme is planned to achieve universal access to health care in South Africa. It is a policy priority. The national budget review indicated the provision of additional funds on health accounts to cover NHI. However, there is a need to present the programme effectively to the public for the average citizen to have a feeling of control. It is portrayed as a financial system designed to source funds for the provision of health care services to all citizens and this has made promoting the plan tricky. This is because the majority of the population use public health services while very few have access to medical aid insurance.

The support for this programme will no doubt increase if the plan is communicated and executed efficiently. Public knowledge about NHI is deficient and based on negative sentiments made openly by those who oppose it (Welthagen, 2019). However, NHI is a reality for developed nations with the success of the programme recorded in Sweden and Germany. As a result, this programme can be said to be of high political importance and low political conflict, as illustrated in Table 10.2 below.

Table 10.2 *Political importance and conflict of NHI in South Africa*

		Conflict	
		Low	High
Political	High	X	
importance	Low		

NHI is about fairness and social protection, and it reflects the type of society that South Africa should strive to be: one that values justice, fairness and social solidarity. The NHI programme is based on the idea that all South Africans, regardless of socioeconomic status, should have access to necessary, high-quality health care services that are provided at no cost. This would protect the population and households from financial difficulties caused by the use of health care services. Vulnerable groups would be given priority. The South African health system has a history of inequity and fragmentation and has been characterized as a two-tiered system with public and private health care providers. South Africa spends around 8.6% of its GDP on health care, which is similar to that of other middle-income countries. However, 84% of the population is uninsured and is handled by an overburdened public health system, while 4.4% of GDP is spent on the 16% of the population who are covered by private medical schemes and who, for the most part, get their health care services in the private sector. Aside from financial resource discrepancy, the health system is marked by human resource maldistribution, with a large share of health care professionals working in the private sector relative to the population. This occurs in the context of a rising disease burden owing to communicable and non-communicable diseases, high maternal and child mortality, and trauma and injuries.

NHI aims to bring South Africa nearer to universal health coverage, in which the entire population, particularly vulnerable populations, is covered; everyone has access to needed quality health services; and households are protected from financial risks and out-of-pocket payments when obtaining health care services, resulting in a unified health system. The NHI programme aims to revolutionize the financing, purchasing and delivery of health care services, based on the requirements of Section 27 of the Bill of Rights, which calls for the progressive realization of the right to health. The NHI is being implemented in three stages over a period of 14 years, which started in 2012, by the National Department of Health. The first phase was implemented between 2012/2013 and 2016/2017. It involved piloting several schemes in readiness for the implementation of the full NHI. Also, workstreams were created to improve the policy and feed in recommendations from the phased implementations. One district was selected in every province in the country apart from Kwazulu-Natal, where two districts were selected, to serve as NHI Pilot districts. The 10 pilot districts were proposed as the location for innovation and testing all through the execution of the first phase of NHI (Setswe, 2020). The operations at this phase were:

(1) ward-based primary health outreach teams (WBPHCOTs) targeted to promote preventive health care to households;

(2) the integrated school health programme (ISHP) aimed at providing health promotion services for school-age children at their schools;

(3) general practitioner (GP) contracting to increase the number of GPs at primary health care (PHC) facilities for improved quality and acceptability of care;

(4) the ideal clinic realization and maintenance model (ICRM) which involved creating minimum standards to increase the quality of services;

(5) district clinical specialist teams (DCST) to aid clinical governance and carry out clinical work, research and training;

(6) centralized chronic medicine dispensing and distribution (CCMDD) to enhance the delivery of medicines, including chronic medication, to patients at pick-up points nearest to the communities;

(7) the health patient registration systems (HPRS) started with capturing patient data and the generation of electronic files but with the ultimate goal of a fully electronic patient record system;

(8) a stock visibility system (SVS) to improve stock lapse using an electronic stock monitoring system to ensure appropriate and timely ordering;

(9) infrastructure projects implemented to improve health infrastructure to ensure increased access and quality of care; and

(10) a workload indicator for staffing needs (WISN), a WHO planning tool intended to help facility managers make more efficient staffing decisions.

Phase 2 (2018–2022) was intended to identify interventions that worked in phase 1 and expand them across provinces and facilities. It focuses on developing the legislation currently in progress. It involves systems and process development for effective management of the NHI Fund. Improvements for this phase (Table 10.3) are found in the financing, health service provision, governance and regulation sectors (NdoH, 2019).

Phase 3 (2023–2026) will expand the health systems and reinforce their activities to full scale. It will involve the introduction of the compulsory prepayment for the NHI, engaging accredited private hospital and specialist services, finalization and implementation of the Medical Schemes Act and NHI Act.

10.4.1   Evaluation of NHI Phase 1

The evaluation for phase 1 was done from November 2017 to December 2018 by a consortium in the country led by Genesis Analytics. The phase was focused on consolidating the health systems. The evaluation report according to the Consortium revealed that there were both challenges and successes (Writer, 2021). All the projects were successful but there were some recommendations, although it was difficult to measure the overall impact of the intervention on access to and quality of services owing to some factors.

Findings from the evaluation revealed the significance of leadership and good governance. This is evident in some of the interventions where committed leaders who embraced the vision of NHI ensured vigorous implementation. The lessons learned from phase 1 will be incorporated into the phase 2 intervention. Notwithstanding, the implementation has been successful in reducing inequality.

10.5   Discussion, conclusion and outlook

Socioeconomic status is related to health outcomes. One area that suffers from inadequacy or deprivation of another aspect of life is health. Studies have shown that inequalities in socioeconomic status are the root cause of health inequalities (Harper & Lynch, 2007; NdoH, 2019). The development of NHI in South Africa is aimed to level out the inequities in public health care by promoting access to health care amongst all South Africans without affordability as a concern.

Table 10.3 *Areas of improvement in the Phase 2 implementation*

Sector	Areas of operation			
	Financing	Provision	Governance	Regulatory
Public sector	(1) Restructuring equitable share (2) Establish a cost-based budget and introduce a case-mix-based budget for hospitals (3) Establish clinic budget and introduce capitation contracting for primary health care (PHC)	(1) School health, maternal and women's health (2) Mental illness, elderly, disability and rehabilitation (3) Expansion of service benefits, and implementation of PHC services through the first 1 000 clinics	(1) Establish central hospitals as semi-autonomous structures (2) Strengthen governance and delegations of hospitals (3) Strengthen governance and delegation of districts	(1) Legislation to create NHI Fund – the NHI Bill introduction (2) Legislation amendments: (i) National Health Act; (ii) The Health Professions Act; (iii) General legislation amendment
Private sector	(1) High price for health services (2) Price regulation for all the services included in the NHI comprehensive benefits framework	(1) Introduction of single service benefits framework (2) Reduce the number of options per scheme	(1) Governance and non-health care (2) Reserves and solvency	(1) Medical Schemes Act and regulations reform

| | Areas of operation | | | |
Sector	Financing	Provision	Governance	Regulatory
	(3) Removal of differential pricing of services based on diagnosis. Copayments and balanced billing.	(3) Reform of PMBs and alignment to NHI services benefits, including common protocols/care pathways		(2) Consolidation: (i) consolidate GEMS and other state medical schemes into a single structure; (ii) reduce the number of medical schemes; (iii) reduce the number of options in medical schemes (3) Licensing of health establishments
Interim institutional structure			(1) Establishment of NHI transitional structures (2) Establishments of health system reform structures (3) Interim NHI fund	

Source: https://businesstech.co.za/news/finance/487827/south-africa-prepares-for-next-phase-of-the-nhi-which-includes-mandatory-pre-payment/

The National Health Act will result in the patient being viewed as a consumer from a legal perspective. Health care will be treated as a commodity, although this may result in the replacement of professional ethics with business ethics; this is evident from current practice in the private sector where doctors are paid on a fee-for-service basis. Some crooked doctors have been caught claiming from the medical insurance company more than once for a particular service rendered to a patient. Also, patients may abuse their autonomy by not following the doctor's advice given to them to help improve their health and this may lead to a waste of resources whereby the same ailment is treated repeatedly.

The NHI will be adopting a capitation method of payment which is based on the number of services offered by the doctor. This may motivate the doctor to over-service to generate more income, thereby becoming solely business-minded at the expense of their patients' health. To reach the target they set for themselves per day, the quality of health care that will be given to their patients may be poor, and this may lead to mis-diagnosis and misinterpretation of patients' health complaints, which will result in poor health outcomes in the country. However, evidence from the implemented phase, as shown in Table 10.4, indicates that the programme is promising in terms of bringing South Africa closer to equality. Inequity in the private and public health services in terms of public health system burden, health care human resources, and financial disparities are beginning to fade, and patients now perceive an improvement in the quality of care as a result of the presence of general practitioners in the public sector. Aside from this, the operations in phase 1 in a way affect other SDGs, aside from aiming for universal health coverage. Objectives 5, 7, 8 and 9 also address SDG9, research and development, through advancing stock monitoring systems, clinical research and training, electronic patient record systems, and improving infrastructures.

A high level of organization and health service coordination is required to achieve the government's goal of a patient-centred, decen-tralized NHI. The time-consuming and extensive processes involved in NHI implementation, such as the allocation of financial and management authority in the DHS, must be taken into account. During the NHI's implementation, the restructuring of public health financing will be critical to its success. However, achieving NHI by 2026 may be impos-sible unless current and future challenges are addressed at the district level. In conclusion, NHI may not be the only solution to the inequality

Table 10.4 *Successes and challenges of NHI Phase 1 interventions*

Intervention	Intervention successes	Intervention challenges
WBPHCOTS	(1) In 2016/2017 a reported 3 519 WBPHCOTs covering 12 816 152 households (2) There was a total of 3 323 WBPHCOTs providing basic health services to children and adults at the end of 2017/2018 (3) These teams were able to successfully fulfill their mandate to provide outreach health services within the community (4) WBPHCOTs did not only complete community visits but they were also able to report on the ill-health or wellbeing of the individuals at the households visited	(1) Team composition was frequently insufficient, with several teams without outreach team leaders (2) The amount of data collected was insufficient to appropriately assess the referral systems and follow-up processes (3) There were occasions when there was insufficient funding for transportation and equipment, which hampered the team's ability to complete their work
ISHP	(1) A total of 4 339 875 learners had been screened through ISHP since 2012, of whom 504 803 were identified as having various health barriers and referred for treatment (2) This intervention is particularly successful in its ability to demonstrate good interdepartmental collaboration between the NDoH and the Department of Basic Education (DBE)	(1) There is a scarcity of data to back up the referrals' success, as well as feedback channels between school teams and facilities (2) Its success was frequently hampered by a lack of adequate equipment, such as measurement scales and transportation to schools (3) During NHI phase 1 execution, there was a lack of prioritization and targeting of learners within this intervention

Table 10.4 *(Cont.)*

Intervention	Intervention successes	Intervention challenges
GP Contracting	(1) A total of 330 GPs had been contracted by end of 2017/2018 (2) Where contracting GPs was implemented successfully, it is evident that access to doctors improved at facilities (3) Patient perception was that the quality of care improved at facilities due to the presence of GPs	(1) Inadequate monitoring of these GPs caused some challenges during implementation (2) Unforeseen contractual challenges during the implementation of this intervention resulted in GPs having substantially higher expense claims than expected
ICRM	(1) A total of 3 434 facilities had been assessed and of these 1 507 had attained ideal clinic status at the end of 2017/2018 (2) ICRM is seen to have improved the ability of facilities to procure much-needed equipment (3) Where ICRM was believed to have been implemented as planned, there was a perceived improvement in the quality of care by both facility managers and patients (4) ICRM limited flexibility and the ability for managers to adapt it to the local context and to the needs of the facilities at the time	(1) The changing manual and frequent change of standards made it difficult for managers to keep up and resulted in frustration among them (2) ICRM offered limited flexibility and limited ability for managers to adapt it to the local context and the needs of the facilities at the time

Table 10.4 *(Cont.)*

Intervention	Intervention successes	Intervention challenges
DCST	(1) At the end of March 2017, 45 of 52 districts in nine provinces had functional DCSTs with at least three members per team (2) The DCSTs, where available, were able to provide specialist oversight within the districts (3) The introduction of these teams was perceived by some stakeholders to have promoted clinical governance within the districts	(1) The team composition, which often lacked critical specialists, limited their ability to provide the envisioned training and support structures (2) The lack of gynaecologists and paediatricians meant that DCSTs were not able to adequately improve child and maternal health as envisioned (3) Not all specialists are necessarily good mentors and may be unable to provide adequate support (4) The DCST model is costly and stretches the limited specialist resources in the public sector
CCMDD	(1) A total of 2 182 422 patients enrolled on the CCMDD, collecting medicines in over 855 PUPs at the end of 2017/2018 (2) The strong political leadership and will behind CCMDD contributed to its successful implementation (3) CCMDD was scaled up beyond the target and the consistent monitoring of the programme contributed to the availability of reliable data to support continued implementation	(1) The change of service providers threatened the intervention's continuity (2) The lack of sufficient integration between CCMDD pick-up points and facilities resulted in inadequate tracking of patients between the two systems

Table 10.4 *(Cont.)*

Intervention	Intervention successes	Intervention challenges
HPRS	(1) At the end of 2017/2018, 2 968 PHC facilities were using HPRS and there were over 20 million (20 700 149) people registered on the system (2) Good communication and feedback loops are seen to have facilitated implementation success	(1) Poor connectivity at some facilities and problems with hardware have contributed to the challenges experienced during NHI phase 1 implementation (2) The lack of human resources and lack of capacity to implement affected the success of HPRS
SVS	(1) At the end of 2017/2018, SVS was being implemented in 3 167 clinics and community health centres (92% coverage) (2) The successful training of available staff led to an in-depth understanding of the system at the facility level (3) The introduction of SVS led to reduced stockouts and improved efficiency at facilities	(1) Lack of reliable internet connectivity and hardware impacted its success (2) The minimal number of available pharmacists and pharmacy assistants limited the facility's ability to ensure the smooth running of the system (3) The sustainability of this intervention poses a challenge as implementation during the NHI phase1 relied heavily on support from external funders
Infrastructure	(1) Since 2013/2014, work in 139 of 140 identified CHCs and clinics has been completed through the NHI rehabilitation projects (2) In 2017/2018 alone, 107 facilities were maintained, repaired and/or refurbished in NHI districts (3) Where completed, patients perceived an improvement in the quality of care as a result (4) Small infrastructure changes had a positive impact on the overall environment at facilities	(1) Projects were rarely implemented or completed due to the lack of planning capacity to release the assigned funds (2) Funds that were released were used mainly for new infrastructure projects and insufficient attention was paid to the maintenance of facilities, which is critical to both access and the provision of quality services and preventing unnecessary new build costs due to deterioration because of a lack of basic maintenance

Table 10.4 *(Cont.)*

Intervention	Intervention successes	Intervention challenges
Human Resources for Health	(1) The introduction of WISN provided a standardized, evidence-based staffing needs assessment at the facility level (2) These assessments were implemented widely across the pilot districts	(1) The resource-constrained environment meant that the hiring of staff had been frozen and, as a result, the WISN findings were not always implementable and caused further frustration among facility managers who had done the assessments

Source: Evaluation of phase 1 implementation of interventions in the National Health Insurance (NHI) pilot districts in South Africa. NDOH10/2017–2018 Final Evaluation Report July 2019

crises in South Africa. There are lots of situations to be tackled, such as unemployment, informal housing, family structure and education. NHI may reduce inequality and inequity in health care but largely the problem that needs to be solved is socioeconomic inequality given the social and economic disparities among the population groups in the country.

References

Ataguba J (2010). Health care financing in South Africa: moving towards universal coverage. Contin Med Educ, 28(2).

Ataguba JE, Akazili J, McIntyre D (2011). Socioeconomic-related health inequality in South Africa: evidence from General Household Surveys. Int J Equity Health, 10:48.

Coovadia H et al. (2009). The health and health system of South Africa: historical roots of current public health challenges. Lancet, 374(9692):817–834.

Fogel R (2019). Informal housing, poverty, and legacies of apartheid in South Africa. Urban@UW: University of Washington | Seattle, WA.

Gilson L et al. (2007). Challenging inequity through health systems. Final report of the Knowledge Network on Health Systems, WHO Commission on the Social Determinants of Health. Geneva: World Health Organization.

Harper S, Lynch J (2007). Trends in socioeconomic inequalities in adult health behaviors among U.S. states, 1990–2004. Public Health Rep, 122(2):177–189.

Harris B et al. (2011). Inequities in access to health care in South Africa. J Public Health Policy, 22(Suppl 1):S102–S123.

IMF (2020). Six Charts Explain South Africa's Inequality. International Monetary Fund.

Mabaso M et al. (2019). HIV prevalence in South Africa through gender and racial lenses: results from the 2012 population-based national household survey. Int J Equity Health, 18(1):167.

Mkhize Z (2019). Opening address by Minister of Health, in National Conference of the Health Professions Council of South Africa. South Africa.

Mohamed S (2021). Failing to learn the lessons? The impact of COVID-19 on a broken and unequal education system. London: Amnesty International.

National Health Insurance Bill (2019). Government Gazette no. 42598.

NdoH (2019). Evaluation of Phase 1 implementation of interventions in the National Health Insurance (NHI) pilot districts in South Africa, Evaluation Report, Final. NDOH10/2017–2018. Johannesburg: Genesis Analytics.

Ojoniyi OO et al. (2019). Does education offset the effect of maternal disadvantage on childhood anemia in Tanzania? Evidence from a nationally representative cross-sectional study. BMC Pediatr, 19(1):89.

Onoka CA, Hanson K, Hanefeld J (2015). Towards universal coverage: a policy analysis of the development of the National Health Insurance Scheme in Nigeria. Health Policy Plan, 30(9):1105–1117.

Setswe G (2020). South Africans should mobilize to support the NHI. Public Health. (https://www.auruminstitute.org/component/content/article/30-blog/public-health/112-south-africans-should-mobilise-to-support-the-nhi?Itemid=101)

Sia D et al. (2014). What lies behind gender inequalities in HIV/AIDS in sub-Saharan African countries: evidence from Kenya, Lesotho, and Tanzania. Health Policy Plan, 29(7):938–949.

UN (2019). Voluntary National Review 2019: High-Level Political Forum on Sustainable Development. (https://sustainabledevelopment.un.org/memberstates/southafrica)

Vally Z (2019). Educational Inequality: The Dark Side Of SA's Education System. Daily Vox.

Welthagen N (2019). Healthcare workers' knowledge of, insight into, and opinion of the proposed National Health Insurance. Solidarity Research Movement, Pretoria, South Africa.

Writer S (2021). South Africa prepares for the next phase of the NHI – which includes mandatory pre-payment. BusinessTech.

Zembe YZ et al. (2013). "Money talks, bullshit walks" interrogating notions of consumption and survival sex among young women engaging in transactional sex in post-apartheid South Africa: a qualitative inquiry. Glob Health, 9(1):1–16.

11 | SDG11, sustainable cities and communities: making cities healthy, sustainable, inclusive and resilient through strong health governance

ROSHANAK MEHDIPANAH,
JAMISON KOEMAN

11.1 Introduction

Today, more than half of the world's population lives in urban areas. While cities are projected to continue to grow, they are currently not equipped to accommodate such large populations when faced with rapid urbanization. This rapid urbanization and growth are resulting in greater socioeconomic inequities, air pollution, overcrowding, displacement and overburdened infrastructure, particularly in developing countries (Eckert & Kohler, 2014; Patil, 2014). Sustainable Development Goal 11 (SDG11), titled "Sustainable cities and communities", comes at a critical time to promote and develop cities that are inclusive, safe, resilient and sustainable. With a multisectoral urban governance approach that emphasizes health, cities can expand successfully and equitably while leaving no residents behind.

This chapter provides an overview of the current struggles experienced by cities, and how urban governance driven by health equity can play a critical role in avoiding rapid and unequal urbanization. Our approach recognizes health as an outcome of, and a precursor to, sustainable cities. However, our reliance on the urban governance framework and our commitment to a health equity lens will favour our interpretation of SDG11 towards one where urban planning changes must be implemented to see a resulting change in health and health equity (Borrell et al., 2013). This chapter will also provide a causal pathway that models the relationship between SDG11 (sustainable cities and communities) and SDG3 (good health and wellbeing) within the context of the other SDGs. For example, the causal pathway will show that SDG2 (zero hunger) mediates the relationship between SDG11 and

SDG3 because access to food is influenced by the urban environment and ultimately impacts people's health. The causal pathway described will show bidirectional arrows due to the complex nature of the interactions. To demonstrate these relationships, we will provide examples of interventions that have been implemented through a multisectoral approach, using urban planning strategies to impact health.

First, the Youth at a Healthy Weight (JOGG) initiative in the Netherlands is a public–private partnership that uses urban planning principles to promote healthy lifestyles for children in municipalities across the Netherlands (JOGG-Aanpak, n.d.). As a response to projections for rising overweight and obesity in the Netherlands, JOGG has grown into a national intervention that has now been implemented in over half of the Netherlands' 352 municipalities. The goal of the intervention is to promote healthy weight in the Netherlands to prevent illness and social costs associated with overweight and obesity. Second, the Barcelona Superblocks in Spain is a large-scale multisectoral initiative that aims to improve public spaces, promote more sustainable mobility, and increase urban green spaces (Palència et al., 2020; Rueda, 2016). Through such programmes, the goal is to address Barcelona's high air pollution levels, reduce noise exposure and traffic injuries, and improve health, culture and economic gains.

Both programmes provide insight on the intersections between urban governance and health system governance and examine their population-health impacts. We use the term *urban governance*, defined as the political power exercised over the physical and social environments within diverse settings and across unequal contexts (Borrell et al., 2013). We refer to *health systems* as the network of public and private institutions that promote health as a primary goal of its function (Agency for Healthcare Research and Quality, 2017). Using this definition and focus on urban areas, we use the term *health system governance* to refer to city-level health systems' power over the physical and social environment within diverse settings and across unequal contexts. Although some of this power may be governed by a national-level health system, implementation of policies and programmes can still differ across cities (WHO, 1991). While both of our main case studies come from high-income settings in Europe, these are strong cases that address some of the consequences of rapid urbanization and provide insight on opportunities that urban health system governance can achieve in developing healthy, sustainable, inclusive and resilient cities.

11.2 Background

As cities continue to grow, it is expected that by 2030, more than 60% of the world's population will be living within an urban area (United Nations Department of Economic and Social Affairs, 2018). The focus is now on how current physical and social environments can accommodate this expanding population. To add to the complexities of overcrowding in many urban areas worldwide, growing socioeconomic inequities will result in a new set of challenges. In particular, cities experiencing fast growth rates have adjusted through rapid urbanization, resulting in swift actions that tend to leave marginalized populations behind. For example, due to a lack of affordable housing, there has been an increase in slum dwellings, and as a result of older infrastructure, water and sanitation systems have been overburdened, resulting in greater periods of shut-offs and sewage-related complications (United Nations, n.d.-b). Furthermore, this unplanned urban sprawl has contributed to greater traffic, directly impacting air and noise pollution in many cities (United Nations, n.d.-a). In 2016, it was estimated that air pollution had caused 4.2 million premature deaths (United Nations Department of Economic and Social Affairs, n.d.).

The disciplines of urban planning and health have long been interconnected (Kochtitzky et al., 2006). Public health and urban planning collaborations date back to the eighteenth and nineteenth centuries when the first wave of migration to cities occurred as a result of growing industrial cities in places like the United Kingdom and the United States (Barton, 2005; Northridge & Freeman, 2011). With this growth, issues of overcrowding and unsanitary conditions began to rise and both sectors came together to address them through more adequate housing and the development of sewage systems. However, as city funding decreased post-industrialization, urban planning became a profitable sector through private development, and public health turned to issues of contagion. Today, the effects of dissociation have become evident with growing evidence of health inequities in cities worldwide. Place-based research has shown the inequities in accessing resources including health, food and social services, primarily in low-income neighbourhoods. These same neighbourhoods are associated with poorer health and life opportunities including education and employment (Ross & Mirowsky, 2001).

SDG11, sustainable cities and communities, comes at a critical time as it recognizes the challenges faced by rapid urbanization. The United

Nations outlines seven targets to better grasp the scope of SDG11 and focus action on the greatest needs. The targets include goals to 1) provide everyone access to an affordable home and basic services, 2) ensure access to affordable transportation, 3) improve urban planning in every country, 4) conserve cultural and natural heritage, 5) reduce deaths by improving disaster responses, 6) reduce the adverse environmental impact of cities, and 7) ensure access to public green space (United Nations, n.d.-a). Investments in infrastructure, public transportation and green spaces can have tremendous benefits for economic activity, climate change and ultimately the health and wellbeing of residents. By developing sustainable cities and communities, we provide opportunities for healthy cities to flourish where they can engage residents and policymakers to address inequities and promote health and wellbeing. Therefore, urban health systems have a critical role to lead, promote and implement good governance and leadership for cities to achieve health and wellbeing.

11.3   Causal pathways

Our framework to identify health policy co-benefits between SDG3 and SDG11 draws on the framework for urban governance outlined by Borrell and colleagues (2013). As shown in Fig. 11.1, health system governance in urban areas influences the urban physical and social environment by providing or influencing the infrastructure needed to perform medical interventions, encourage healthy behaviours, and improve resource access (WHO, 1991). For instance, the health system may combine urban planning, the natural environment and environmental characteristics to create green spaces that help reduce the health impacts of air pollution while creating opportunities for residents to exercise, play and relax. However, health system intervention in the urban environment is not always equitable. It may result in inequities in access to resources and medical care, across social class, race, ethnicity, gender, sexuality, ability and age dimensions. For example, while health systems may determine the location of health care facilities throughout a city, without adequate public transportation, some residents, particularly those with no access to private vehicles, may not be able to access those services. Urban inequities lead to population health inequities and exacerbate population health needs, which

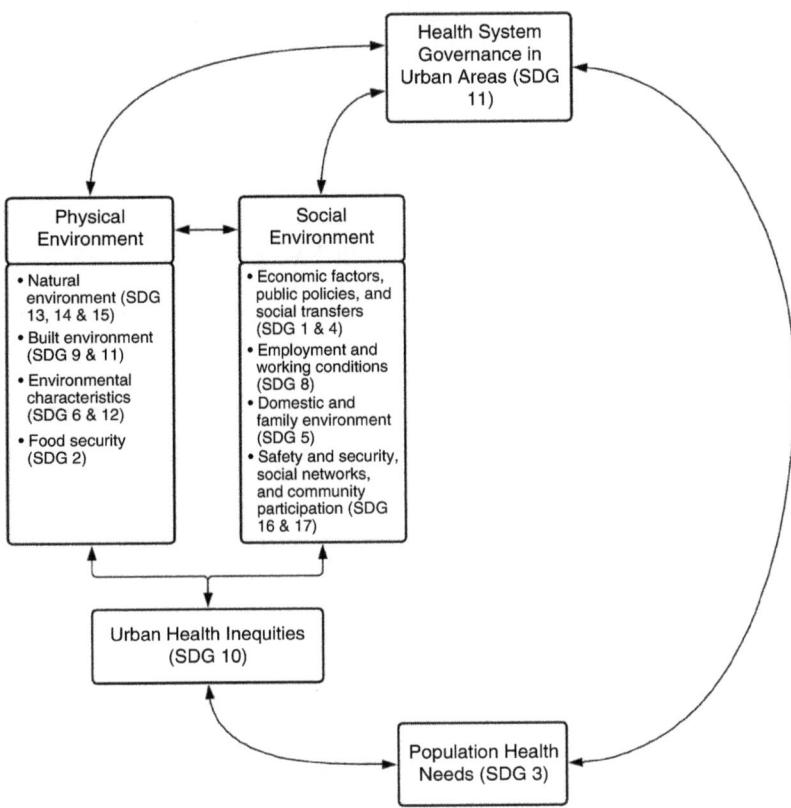

Fig. 11.1 Urban health system governance and Sustainable Development Goal co-benefits

therefore influence and dictate how health systems should govern the urban environment. These inequities are attributed to historical and contemporary policies that result in the segregation of residents based on social class, race and ethnicity (Dwyer, 2010; Taeuber & Taeuber, 2009). Segregated areas are then more susceptible to disinvestment and lack of resources that directly impact the health of residents (Acevedo-Garcia & Lochner, 2003). For instance, many cities failed to equitably distribute the COVID-19 vaccine, resulting in population health needs specific to certain groups (DiRago et al., 2022). Box 11.1 describes the example of Chicago.

Box 11.1 Unequal vaccination in Chicago, USA

In cities where COVID-19 vaccines have become available, vaccine distribution has been inequitable, contributing to unequal COVID-19 infections, hospitalizations and deaths. The Chicago Health Department collected in-depth data on COVID-19 infections, hospitalizations and deaths by race throughout the pandemic and it demonstrates the inequity in vaccination. In the earliest stages of COVID-19 vaccine rollout in Chicago, vaccines were disproportionately administered to White Chicagoans. Even though 33% of Chicago residents are White and 59% are Black or Latinx, in the first week of vaccine rollout over 65% of the vaccines were administered to White Chicagoans compared to 18% for Black and Latinx Chicagoans (Chicago Department of Public Health, n.d.). As of 25 June 2021, in Chicago, six months after the first doses were administered, inequities still persisted as 38% of the Black population and 46% of the Latinx population had received at least one dose of the vaccine compared to 61% of the White population (Chicago Department of Public Health, n.d.).

Inequitable vaccination translated to inequitable health impacts (Zeng et al., 2021). The June 25th Reopening Metrics Update showed that Black and Latinx Chicagoans represented a far larger portion of COVID-19 cases, hospitalizations and deaths, compared to White and Asian Chicagoans. Black and Latinx Chicagoans were represented in about 75% of COVID-19 cases from 19 June to 25 June 2021, greater than three out of every four COVID-19 hospitalizations from 1 June to 25 June, and greater than three of every four COVID-19 deaths in the city of Chicago from 1 May to 22 June 2021 (Chicago Department of Public Health, 2021). These massive racial gaps in COVID-19 health outcomes should indicate to Chicago health authorities the need to prioritize reaching the Black and Latinx populations in COVID-19 interventions moving forward.

There is a strong relationship between SDG3 and SDG11, as health system governance in urban areas is linked to the urban planning and public policy sectors. Population health is directly and indirectly impacted by physical and social factors like city infrastructure, land costs, property taxes, transportation and housing. Providing health services in a sustainable city requires a built environment that includes buildings to house health services and community amenities like food outlets and green spaces to promote public health. Health services practitioners have outlined that the provision of health services should involve an accessible location; design principles that create a patient-friendly, healing, spacious, clean, flexible and accommodating environment; and amenities located in the surrounding environment that provide food, shopping, internet access and childcare services (Luxon, 2015). The principle of accessibility is especially important for promoting urban health equity. For example, during the COVID-19 pandemic, people with mobility and cognitive impairments saw impacts on their caregiving and more barriers in accessing care owing to limited accommodating public policies (Baumer, 2021; Landes et al., 2020; Turk et al., 2020). Furthermore, social distancing policies resulted in disruptions in care and isolation, while lack of utilities including water and electricity made it difficult for many to stay at home (Pineda & Corburn, 2020).

As health systems alter physical and social environments in urban areas, they will influence other SDGs. For instance, a health system that prioritizes green space to give city residents an outdoor space for exercise, games and sports will produce co-benefits for SDG15 (Life on land) by providing a place for plants and animals to live and grow. Health system governance in urban areas can also have a co-benefit with SDG1 (no poverty), SDG2 (zero hunger), SDG4 (quality education) and SDG8 (decent work and economic growth) by stimulating economic activity and investment. For example, hospitals can serve as important "anchor institutions" that contribute to the vitality of the surrounding urban area (Schwartz, 2017). Globally, about 60 per 10 000 people are medical doctors or nurses (WHO, 2021). In the United States, the country that spends the most on health care, the health care sector employs about one in eight jobs (KFF, 2021). Additional jobs are supported indirectly, through purchase of goods and services from other businesses (American Hospital Association, 2017).

In addition, the health care sectors of wealthier countries are beginning to address social needs arising from health inequities associated with the physical and social environments in growing urban areas. In the United Kingdom, a model known as "social prescribing" links patients of primary care physicians to social and community services to improve health, wellbeing and social connection (Bickerdike et al., 2017). Interventions typically involve link workers, who connect patients to resources such as housing, welfare and budgeting, education and literacy, peer networks, counselling, exercise activities, outdoor recreation, gardening and others (Tierney et al., 2020). For example, Life Rooms, a social prescribing intervention for people with mental illness who reside in disadvantaged communities in Liverpool and Sefton (UK), connects patients with learning opportunities and financial counselling (Hassan et al., 2020). In the United States, non-profit hospitals are required to perform community investment in order to maintain their tax-exempt status. As a result, a growing number of hospitals are implementing interventions that reconstruct and influence the physical and social environments and opportunities surrounding patients, including creating affordable housing, promoting nutritious food access, expanding transportation options, enhancing local education, and constructing community facilities (Horwitz et al., 2020; Koeman & Mehdipanah, 2021; Schwartz, 2017).

However, we return to equity as a key priority for health systems, since a health system's outreach and intervention within an area may have the unintended consequence of contributing towards gentrification in cities by increasing property values and "pricing out" the surrounding community (Box 11.2) (Cole et al., 2021). Academic scholarship has debated the comparative strength and influence of the public and private sectors in the health system and their potential impacts on urban health

---

Box 11.2 Hospital-caused gentrification in Amman, Jordan

In Amman, Jordan, the development of two hospitals highlights the detrimental consequences for urban areas that can occur when little coordination goes into the development of a private hospital. Jordan Hospital is a 247-bed hospital that was initiated in 1996 and Khalidi Hospital is a 160-bed hospital that was initiated in 1978. At the time that these hospitals were built, private hospitals were subject to very few requirements and regulations regarding city planning and the locations of the hospitals were largely subject to the population's medical needs and city's circumstances. Private hospitals saw an opportunity for profit owing to the location and health services demand, city laws allowed for an easy change from residential to commercial zoning, and no city-wide planning went into the development of these two hospitals. As a result, the introduction of these two private hospitals increased land prices and dramatically changed the composition of the surrounding area, increasing the number of commercial and medical buildings while decreasing the number of residential buildings including affordable housing. The changes also resulted in more traffic jams and little space for parking in the areas surrounding the two hospitals (Irmeili & Sharaf, 2017).

equity. Research has suggested that health systems with a greater reliance on the private sector may place less emphasis on equity, public health and primary care and will be less coordinated than those with a greater reliance on the public sector (Basu et al., 2012). This is evident in a growing body of research that discusses health care gentrification where for-profit health care systems favour wealthier residents by situating themselves in higher-income areas, including areas recently gentrified, to improve profit returns as opposed to reducing health care inequalities (Dahrouge et al., 2018; Martínez et al., 2016; Sumah, Baatiema & Abimbola, 2016). Regardless of whether the public or private sector is dominant, more investment in policies and regulations focusing on zoning and land development are needed to promote health across the whole city and improve the sustainability of the urban health system (Elsey et al., 2019).

11.4 Case study 1: Youth at a Healthy Weight (JOGG) initiative in Dutch cities

Our first case study describes the Youth at a Healthy Weight (Jongeren op Gezond Gewicht – JOGG) intervention in the Netherlands. JOGG is a national organization with ANBI status (non-profit) that promotes public–private partnership between the Netherlands Ministry of Health, Welfare and Sport, local municipalities and private partners to improve healthy living for youth in the Netherlands by altering the urban physical and social environments. The focus on the environment surrounding youth mirrors the EPODE approach, a methodology established in France and in use in similar projects in six European countries (Borys et al., 2012). JOGG was established in 2014 out of the efforts of the Healthy Weight Covenant and has since cultivated a diverse network of partners that now includes the Netherlands Ministry of Health, Welfare and Sport, over 180 municipalities and nearly 40 other organizations (Collard et al., 2019; JOGG-Aanpak, n.d.; Renders et al., 2010). Early developments in JOGG's network building included partnering with six business partners to focus on promoting good nutrition and exercise, but quickly developed into a national effort (Slot-Heijs et al., 2020). In 2018, JOGG signed the National Prevention Agreement, elevating its role in promoting a healthier Netherlands (Ministry of Health, Welfare and Sport, 2019). With 90% of funding coming from the Ministry of Health, Welfare and Sport, JOGG is now a national organization that recommends and helps municipalities implement strategies (Slot-Heijs et al., 2020).

Between 2015 and 2019, JOGG expanded in four important ways. First, the amount of funding that JOGG received from the Ministry of Health, Welfare and Sport almost doubled between 2015 and 2019, from $3.9 million to $7.6 million. Second, the number of social partners grew from 16 in 2015 to 22 in 2019 and the number of business partners grew from 6 in 2015 to 14 in 2019. Third, the number of municipalities partnering with JOGG (JOGG municipalities) grew from 91 in 2015 to 143 in 2019. As a result, the number of children and youth living in JOGG municipalities grew from 545 243 in 2015 to 1 195 111 in 2019, a number that represents nearly half of the country's youth population. Finally, the percentage of JOGG municipalities that have appointed a JOGG director for at least 16 hours per week grew from 41% in 2015 to 81% in 2019 (Slot-Heijs et al., 2020).

JOGG's growth results from the Netherlands' response to an alarming outlook that projected an increase in adult overweight and obesity. According to the Netherlands Public Health Future Outlook, the percentage of overweight Dutch adults will rise from 49% in 2015 to 62% in 2040 (National Institute for Public Health and the Environment, 2018). Rising overweight and obesity is especially alarming because of a resulting impact on social costs. For example, rising overweight and obesity contributed to 3.7% of the burden of disease and €1.5 billion in health care costs in the Netherlands in 2018 (Gibson et al., 2017; National Institute for Public Health and the Environment, 2018; Quek et al., 2017). As a result, the 2018 Dutch National Prevention Agreement, which JOGG signed, highlighted overweight and obesity in order to reverse these trends (Ministry of Health, Welfare and Sport, 2019). Furthermore, JOGG decided that the Netherlands' youth population is an appropriate area to intervene because 13.2% of children aged 4 to 18 years in the Netherlands were overweight or obese in 2018 (National Institute for Public Health and the Environment, 2018).

The "JOGG approach" connects stakeholders and intervenes in living environments to promote health among people younger than 19 years old (JOGG-Aanpak, n.d.). Because the focus is to improve health by altering the physical and social environments around youth, the JOGG approach exemplifies the potential for co-benefit between SDG3 and SDG11. The JOGG approach addresses seven environments that children and youth contact the most: home, neighbourhood, school, sport, leisure, work and media (JOGG-Aanpak, n.d.). Several of these environments correspond closely to the physical and social environments described in the Urban Health System Governance Framework (Fig. 11.1). For example, home and neighbourhood, key intervention environments, are part of the built environment (SDG11). In the city of Eindhoven, JOGG partnered with Ballast Nedam Development, a private developer, to promote healthy urbanization on the Berckelbosch development project (Ballast Nedam Development, 2020). The Berckelbosch development project involves the development of 950 homes in Eindhoven and the partnership with JOGG involves creating a healthier urban environment with ample green space, safe walking and biking, and infrastructure for sports and games (Berckelbosch Eindhoven, n.d.).

Preliminary results suggest that the JOGG approach improves health (SDG3) and promotes health equity (SDG10). While two studies conflict in their analysis of the overweight prevalence in children between JOGG and non-JOGG areas, both show an overall decrease in overweight prevalence of almost 10% in JOGG areas over the study period (Kobes, Kretschmer & Timmerman, 2021; National Institute for Public Health and the Environment, 2020). However, this result must be interpreted with caution. The studies do not rule out the possibility that decreases in overweight and obesity were happening before JOGG was implemented, that other initiatives may be more responsible for the decrease, or that relevant differences between municipalities skew the results (National Institute for Public Health and the Environment, 2020). In fact, one study concluded that it is socioeconomic status (SES) that most likely explains this result, not the approach's success. Yet when analysing only low SES areas that implemented JOGG at least six years ago, which were typically areas with the highest overweight prevalence, this study showed a significant decrease in overweight prevalence, suggesting that JOGG is especially successful in the areas most severely affected by overweight and obesity (Kobes, Kretschmer & Timmerman, 2021). The preliminary results suggest that JOGG improves health in some areas (SDG3) and the unequal reach of the intervention is moving in a positive direction, where low SES areas are more strongly benefited, thereby promoting health equity across Dutch municipalities. According to the Health System Governance Framework (Fig. 11.1), this is a case where the intervention on the physical and social environments alleviates urban health inequities (SDG10).

The JOGG approach has significant potential for co-benefits with other SDGs, which increases its importance. SDGs 4 (Quality education) and 2 (Zero hunger) are two examples. Over 1500 schools work with Healthy School, an initiative funded in part by JOGG (JOGG-Aanpak, n.d.). Healthy School is a national collaboration between several ministries that have developed a step-by-step plan for promoting an educational environment that helps children thrive. It involves four pillars: education to develop skills needed for a healthy lifestyle; a school environment that helps children pursue a healthy lifestyle; identification of health problems at an early age; and incorporation of health promotion measures into school policy (Gezonde School, n.d.). JOGG also used the school environment to address food security (SDG2). Over the 2020–2021 school year, JOGG piloted a programme to improve healthy food in schools in the cities of Alkmaar, Lelystad and Katwijk. The pilot was focused on limiting an unhealthy food supply in the municipality, making the food supply around schools healthier, and influencing healthy choices within schools (JOGG, 2021).

The Intersectoral Governance Framework (Table 11.1) describes the tools and actions JOGG used to produce co-benefits between SDG11 and SDG3. The table reflects organizational shifts from the Dutch National Prevention Agreement, intervention through civic engagement, and accountability through evaluation. First, along with the Ministry of Health, Welfare and Sport and various social partners, JOGG helped to develop and signed the National Prevention Agreement in 2018, which committed JOGG and its partners to a coordinated plan, increased JOGG's funding, set its goals and targets, identified shared objectives across partners and ministries, and altered its organizational structure. In 2019, 90% of JOGG's $8.5 million budget was funded by the Ministry of Health, Welfare and Sport (Slot-Heijs et al., 2020). The National Prevention Agreement created the target and indicator to reduce youth overweight and obesity prevalence to 9.1% and 2.3% respectively by 2040 (Ministry of Health, Welfare and Sport, 2019). Many of JOGG's business and social partners provided input and signed the agreement, and the agreement identifies shared objectives between ministries. For example, the National Prevention Agreement identifies cycling to school and work as an intervention area, which overlaps with the transportation goals of the Ministry of Infrastructure and Water Management (Ministry of Health, Welfare and Sport, 2019). Also in response to the National Prevention Agreement, JOGG's organizational structure

Table 11.1 *Intersectoral governance framework: the case of JOGG*

			Possible governance actions with these tools								
			Goals and targets	Evidence support	Policy guidance	Implementation and management	Coordination	Advocacy	Monitoring and evaluation	Financial support	Legal mandate
Tools	Plan	Plan				X	X				
	Indicators and targets	Indicators	X						X		
		Targets	X								
	Budgeting	Pooled budget									
		Shared objectives	X				X				
		Coordinated budgeting									
	Organization	Ministerial linkages									
		Specific ministers	X			X				X	
		Organization	X		X	X	X				
		Legislative committees									
		Interdepartmental committees/units									
		Departmental mergers									
		Civic engagement			X	X	X				
	Accountability	Transparent data		X	X				X		
		Regular reporting		X	X				X		X
		Independent agency/evaluators		X	X				X		X
		Support for civil society									
		Legal rights									

changed, obtaining a board of directors and a scientific advisory committee to manage and advise JOGG's progress and evaluation methods. Second, JOGG intervenes through partnership with municipalities and helps them implement local interventions. JOGG municipalities utilize members from the municipality to form a JOGG team that includes a JOGG director, JOGG policy officer and other stakeholders from the municipality in order to promote civic engagement (JOGG-Aanpak, n.d.). As a reflection of local partnership, the Association of Dutch Municipalities, which represents the interests of all Dutch municipalities, also committed to the National Prevention Agreement (Ministry of Health, Welfare and Sport, 2019). Third, JOGG is held accountable through evaluation. The National Prevention Agreement also mandated that the National Institute for Public Health and the Environment, an independent agency, will monitor progress towards the goals in order to guide policy decisions (Ministry of Health, Welfare and Sport, 2019). This agency, in collaboration with the Mulier Institute, has produced annual reports for JOGG since 2015 (Slot-Heijs et al., 2020). JOGG also provides transparent data to document its partnerships and partner municipalities (JOGG-Aanpak, n.d.).

The JOGG approach is favourable on the conflict-political importance scale represented in Table 11.2. The JOGG approach has become more important and less conflictual in the last several years, as indicated by its rapid growth. Continued expansion will indicate the increasing popularity of this intervention. While the intervention is popular, a legal mandate as well as a more active role in coordinating and recommending municipal actions from the national government may improve the intervention's reach. For example, a legal mandate could require all municipalities to meet a set of recommendations in the seven environments that JOGG prioritizes. Further, JOGG must be careful to minimize conflicts of interest among its business and social partners. The

Table 11.2 *Political importance and conflict: the case of JOGG*

		Conflict	
		Low	High
Political importance	High	X	
	Low		

EPODE International Network, of which JOGG is a member, is funded by Nestlé, potentially causing conflicts of interest to arise from food retailers that have an adverse impact on obesity rates (Borys et al., 2012; Cision, 2012). Nevertheless, JOGG is a strong example of an intervention with low political conflict and high political importance that has benefited youth health by emphasizing healthy change to surrounding environments and prioritizing building a strong network of partners.

11.5   Case study 2: Superblocks in Barcelona

Over the last couple of decades, Barcelona has experienced challenges attributed to population growth that have impacted the health and health behaviours of its residents (Agència de Salut Pública, 2021). This has included a rise in environmental hazards including air pollution, while traffic injuries and a lack of green spaces have contributed to rising sedentary behaviours and health complications. At pre-2020 pollution levels (years 2018–2019), it was estimated that in the city of Barcelona 7% of natural deaths (about 1000 deaths per year), about 11% of new cases of lung cancer (about 110 cases per year) and about 33% of new cases of childhood asthma (about 525 cases per year) were attributed to air pollution in excess of WHO recommendations (10 $\mu g/m^3$ PM2.5 and 20 $\mu g/m^3$ NO2) (Rico et al., 2020). In response to these issues and others, in May 2016, the Barcelona city council approved the measure "Omplim de vida els careers" ("Improving life on the streets"), to create Superblocks across the city (Ajuntament de Barcelona, n.d.; Mehdipanah et al., 2019; Rueda, 2016). The Barcelona Superblocks consist of amalgamations of blocks throughout the city to improve the habitability of public spaces, sustainable mobility, and urban green, and to promote residents' participation and co-responsibility (Ajuntament de Barcelona, n.d.). If the initially planned 503 Superblocks were to be implemented, it is estimated that it would reduce annual air pollution by 24% and could prevent almost 700 annual premature deaths (Mueller et al., 2020). Ultimately, the Barcelona Superblock programme aims to achieve the sustainable city and community development goal of SDG11 by improving the physical and social environments within intervened areas (Fig. 11.1).

The Barcelona Superblocks were developed by the Department of Ecology and Infrastructures of the Barcelona city council. Each superblock promotes universal accessibility by redeveloping interior spaces for pedestrians and cyclists while creating more opportunities for public spaces to help facilitate cultural, economic and social exchanges. By reducing speed limits to 10km/h and increasing public spaces, the Superblocks aim to ultimately improve quality of life for residents and create more opportunities for social cohesion and economic activity. At the heart of this intersectoral approach to the Barcelona Superblocks is the participatory process that is meant to be inclusive of residents living within the intervention neighbourhoods. A three-step planning process is undertaken. First, a team from the city's Department of Planning and Prospection and the Management of Urban Model Projects drafts an Action Plan for each designated area. Second, through a participatory process involving neighbourhood associations and residents, each Action Plan is finalized. Third, the Action Plan is implemented. Through a partnership with the Public Health Agency of Barcelona, the Superblocks were evaluated for their effects on the environment, health and health inequities (Agència de Salut Publica, n.d.). Currently, although they are small interventions, five superblocks have been completed, with another three within the implementation process. The goal is to implement Superblocks in each of Barcelona's ten districts.

So far, the initiative has reduced air and noise pollution, promoted more interactions among residents, and some improvements in physical activity (Agència de Salut Publica, n.d.). Although there are still concerns among residents around traffic congestion and safety, the Barcelona Superblocks are an important example of urban governance addressing issues associated with urban growth.

Using the Intersectoral Governance Framework (Table 11.3), planning was used as a tool across all possible governance actions including setting goals and targets, guiding policy and the implementation and management of the programme. Multiple departments are involved throughout the planning, implementation and evaluation phases, including the role of the Barcelona Public Health Agency in assessing the environmental and health impacts of the Superblocks (Mehdipanah et al., 2019; Palència et al., 2020). Central to the Barcelona Superblocks is the public engagement piece that ensures residents provide input on the planning and implementation phases of the projects. Furthermore, residents' opinions are captured through surveys and interviews post-implementation to better understand the perceptions towards multiple aspects of the projects including traffic, public spaces and social networking opportunities. In addition, businesses are also

Table **11.3** *Intersectoral governance framework: the case of the Barcelona Superblocks*

			Possible governance actions with these tools								
			Goals and targets	Evidence support	Policy guidance	Implementation and management	Coordination	Advocacy	Monitoring and evaluation	Financial support	Legal mandate
Tools	Plan	Plan	X	X	X	X	X	X	X	X	X
	Indicators and targets	Indicators	X	X					X		
		Targets	X			X			X		
	Budgeting	Pooled budget								X	
		Shared objectives				X					
		Coordinated budgeting								X	
	Organization	Ministerial linkages	X			X					
		Specific ministers		X					X		
		Organization				X	X				
		Legislative committees									
		Interdepartmental committees/units	X		X	X					
		Departmental mergers									
		Civic engagement	X			X	X				
	Accountability	Transparent data							X		
		Regular reporting							X		
		Independent agency/evaluators							X		
		Support for civil society									
		Legal rights									

Table 11.4 *Political importance and conflict: the case of the Barcelona Superblocks*

		Conflict	
		Low	High
Political importance	High	X	
	Low		

interviewed to better understand the economic gains of these projects through the greater foot traffic and visibility provided.

The Barcelona Superblocks involve multiple players in the funding, development, implementation and evaluation processes. For example, funding came together from pooling and coordinating budgets from the federal and regional governments through initiatives aimed to support public transportation. This illustrates that through the programme's multiple outcomes, including the reduction of environmental hazards and better transportation, the Barcelona Superblocks are well positioned to attract and attain diverse financial support.

On a political importance and conflict scale, the Barcelona Superblock is of high political importance and high conflict (Table 11.4). The Superblock initiative addresses major issues the city faced in relation to air pollution and traffic. Concerns have been raised through residents and community organizations in relation to potential gentrification and displacement, in addition to the unequal distribution of health benefits, particularly in the initial neighbourhoods where residents' input was not considered. Residents have demonstrated both support and opposition (Torres, 2019). At a political level, the initiative has been challenged by the conservative opposition and used to criticize the progressive government of Ada Colau, the current mayor of Barcelona (Klause, 2018).

Nonetheless, sustainability and continued financial investment in such a programme is an imminent concern, particularly when regional or state level governments dictate programme funding. This has been an issue in Barcelona where, in 2011, the Llei de Barris (Neighbourhood Law) urban renewal programme had invested approximately €1.3 billion in improving 143 largely disinvested neighbourhoods throughout the Catalonia region (Departament de Politica Territorial i Obres

Publiques, 2009). While the goal was to continue expanding the programme, in 2012, the newly elected conservative coalition suspended the programme's funding. Although the government made a renewed commitment to complete existing programmes in 2014, disruptions through unfinished programmes had impacted neighbourhood residents and businesses (Mehdipanah et al., 2014).

To prevent similar occurrences, programmes like the Barcelona Superblocks must seek multiple funding sources, including both public and private investments to ensure the continuity of growth. They must also continue working with various sectors to demonstrate the added value the initiative brings, including public health, where a recent evaluation showed the positive effects on health with an improvement in the quality of life of residents and people who used the Superblocks. The reduction in noise, improvement in sleep quality, decrease in air pollution and increase in social interactions were all contributing factors to the improved wellbeing reported by residents (Agència de Salut Publica, n.d.).

11.6   Conclusion

In this chapter we presented a background for understanding the close relationship between urban planning and public health, a framework for understanding the co-benefits between SDG11 and SDG3, and two examples that illustrate health system governance in urban areas. Through this work, two important themes necessary to understand co-benefits between the two SDGs emerged. First, achieving SDG11, that is, making cities healthy, sustainable, inclusive and resilient, is a prerequisite to achieving good health and wellbeing (SDG3). Under the health system governance framework identified in the causal pathways section, we showed that health systems govern through altering the physical and social environment with direct and indirect health impacts. With a growing population living in cities, the importance of SDG11 as a catalyst to achieve good population health and wellbeing cannot be underestimated. As we identified above, green spaces in a city allow for exercise, quality transportation is necessary to acquire resources such as medical care, and vaccine equity is necessary for achieving strong population health. In addition, the JOGG and superblocks interventions suggest that a healthy, sustainable, inclusive and resilient city has potential to improve population health. The JOGG approach targets the environment surrounding a child to promote healthy growth and the superblocks create public spaces that allow for residents to connect. To create co-benefits between SDG3 and SDG11, intervening on SDG11, the built environment around the population, with the goal of improving health is a common and strong approach.

Second, addressing health inequities should be a strong priority in ensuring urban growth is sustainable, inclusive and resilient, and to promote equity, the health system and other urban governance structures must work together to create strong intersectoral collaboration. More equitable policies and practices around land development and zoning can produce more equitable growth, reduce negative impacts of for-profit development, including gentrification, and promote good health and wellbeing (Basu et al., 2012; Dahrouge et al., 2018; Martínez et al., 2016; Sumah et al., 2016). Stronger coordination between public and private, health care and social services, and profit-making and mission-driven sectors in a health system can promote the commitment to equity necessary for sustainable, inclusive and resilient cities. The JOGG and superblocks interventions are excellent examples of interventions that are developing strong intersectoral partnerships. Through partnership with the Ministry of Health, Welfare and Sport, municipalities, business partners and social partners, JOGG has reduced overweight prevalence in low-SES areas, improving health equity in the Netherlands. Using interdepartmental collaboration and public engagement, the superblocks intervention has reduced air and noise pollution, promoted more interactions among residents, and improved physical activity.

As countries look to improve their commitment to building sustainable, healthy, inclusive and resilient cities, stronger coordination across multiple sectors is needed to ensure policies and programmes targeting equitable growth are in place to prevent the negative consequences of rapid urbanization. As the global population continues to shift towards urban living, these areas must provide opportunities for residents to thrive healthfully.

Acknowledgement

We would like to thank Dr Katherine Pérez and the Salut als Carrers Working Group for their guidance on the Barcelona superblocks case study.

References

Acevedo-Garcia D, Lochner KA (2003). Residential Segregation and Health. In: Kawachi I, Berkman LF (eds), Neighborhoods and Health. Oxford University Press. (https://doi.org/10.1093/acprof:oso/9780195138382.003.0012)

Agència de Salut Pública (2021). La salut a Barcelona. ASPB – Agència de Salut Pública de Barcelona. (https://www.aspb.cat/documents/salutbarcelona/)

Agència de Salut Publica (n.d.). Salut als Carrers. Avaluació dels àmbits Superilles. ASPB – Agència de Salut Pública de Barcelona. (https://www.aspb.cat/documents/salutalscarrers/, 8 September 2022)

Agency for Healthcare Research and Quality (2017). Defining Health Systems. (https://www.ahrq.gov/chsp/chsp-reports/resources-for-understanding-health-systems/defining-health-systems.html)

Ajuntament de Barcelona (n.d.). Superblocks—'Let's fill the streets with life' | Ecology. Urban Planning, Infrastructures and Mobility. (https://ajuntament.barcelona.cat/ecologiaurbana/en/bodies-involved/citizen-participation/superblocks, 8 September 2022)

American Hospital Association (2017). Hospitals are Economic Anchors in their Communities. (https://www.aha.org/statistics/2018-03-29-hospitals-are-economic-anchors-their-communities)

Ballast Nedam Development (2020). A first: Ballast Nedam Development and JOGG work together for a healthy physical living environment. (https://www.development.ballast-nedam.nl/nieuws/2020/primeur-ballast-nedam-development-en-jogg-samen-aan-de-slag-voor-een-gezonde-fysieke-leefomgeving/)

Barton H (2005). A Health Map for Urban Planners: Towards a Conceptual Model for Healthy, Sustainable Settlements. Built Environ, 31(4):339–355.

Basu S, Andrews J, Kishore S et al. (2012). Comparative Performance of Private and Public Healthcare Systems in Low- and Middle-Income Countries: A Systematic Review. PLoS Med, 9(6):e1001244. (https://doi.org/10.1371/journal.pmed.1001244)

Baumer N (2021). The pandemic isn't over—Particularly for people with disabilities. Harvard Health. (https://www.health.harvard.edu/blog/the-pandemic-isnt-over-particularly-for-people-with-disabilities-202105252464)

Berckelbosch Eindhoven (n.d.). (https://www.berckelbosch.nl/, 28 June 2021)

Bickerdike L, Booth A, Wilson PM et al. (2017). Social prescribing: Less rhetoric and more reality. A systematic review of the evidence. BMJ Open, 7(4):e013384. (https://doi.org/10.1136/bmjopen-2016-013384)

Borrell C, Pons-Vigués M, Morrison J et al. (2013). Factors and processes influencing health inequalities in urban areas. J Epidemiol Community Health, 67(5):389–391. (https://doi.org/10.1136/jech-2012-202014)

Borys J-M, Le Bodo Y, Jebb SA et al. (2012). EPODE approach for childhood obesity prevention: Methods, progress and international development. Obes Rev, 13(4):299–315. (https://doi.org/10.1111/j.1467-789X.2011.00950.x)

Chicago Department of Public Health (2021). Protecting Chicago: Phase IV Re-Opening Metrics Update. (https://www.chicago.gov/content/city/en/sites/covid-19/home/covid-data-reports.html)

Chicago Department of Public Health (n.d.). Vaccination Data At A Glance. (https://www.chicago.gov/city/en/sites/covid19-vaccine/home/vaccination-data-at-a-glance.html, 28 June 2021)

Cision (2012). EPODE International Network: The Epode European Network is a success story! (https://www.businesswire.com/news/home/20121220005403/en/EPODE-International-Network-The-Epode-European-Network-is-a-success-story%21)

Cole HVS, Mehdipanah R, Gullón P et al. (2021). Breaking Down and Building Up: Gentrification, Its drivers, and Urban Health Inequality. Curr Environ Health Rep, 8(2):157–166. (https://doi.org/10.1007/s40572-021-00309-5)

Collard D, Slot-Heijs J, Dellas V et al. (2019). Monitor Jongeren Op Gezond Gewicht 2018 (1–95). Utrecht. (https://www.kennisbanksportenbewegen.nl/?file=9417&m=1552308391&action=file.download)

Dahrouge S, Hogg W, Muggah E et al. (2018). Equity of primary care service delivery for low income "sicker" adults across 10 OECD countries. Int J Equity Health, 17:182. (https://doi.org/10.1186/s12939-018-0892-z)

Departament de Politica Territorial i Obres Publiques (2009). La Llei de Barris: Una aposta collectiva per la cohesio social. Catalunya.

DiRago NV, Li M, Tom T et al. (2022). COVID-19 Vaccine Rollouts and the Reproduction of Urban Spatial Inequality: Disparities Within Large US Cities in March and April 2021 by Racial/Ethnic and Socioeconomic Composition. J Urban Health, 99(2):191–207. (https://doi.org/10.1007/s11524-021-00589-0)

Dwyer RE (2010). Poverty, Prosperity, and Place: The Shape of Class Segregation in the Age of Extremes. Soc Probl, 57(1):114–137. (https://doi.org/10.1525/sp.2010.57.1.114)

Eckert S, Kohler S (2014). Urbanization and health in developing countries: A systematic review. World Health Popul, 15(1):7–20. (https://doi.org/10.12927/whp.2014.23722)

Elsey H, Agyepong I, Huque R et al. (2019). Rethinking health systems in the context of urbanisation: Challenges from four rapidly urbanising low-income and middle-income countries. BMJ Glob Health, 4(3):e001501. (https://doi.org/10.1136/bmjgh-2019-001501)

Gezonde School (n.d.). What is Healthy School? (https://gezondeschool.nl/aanpak/wat-is-gezonde-school, 30 June 2021)

Gibson LY, Allen KL, Davis E et al. (2017). The psychosocial burden of childhood overweight and obesity: Evidence for persisting difficulties in boys and girls. Eur J Pediatr, 176(7):925–933. (https://doi.org/10.1007/s00431-017-2931-y)

Hassan SM, Giebel C, Morasae EK et al. (2020). Social prescribing for people with mental health needs living in disadvantaged communities: The Life Rooms model. BMC Health Serv Res, 20:19. (https://doi.org/10.1186/s12913-019-4882-7)

Horwitz LI, Chang C, Arcilla HN et al. (2020). Quantifying Health Systems' Investment In Social Determinants Of Health, By Sector, 2017–19. Health Aff (Millwood), 39(2):192–198. (https://doi.org/10.1377/hlthaff.2019.01246)

Irmeili G, Sharaf F (2017). The Impact of Private Hospitals on Surrounding Urban Areas: This Following Case is for Study in Amman. Dev Ctry Stud, 7(1):40–48.

JOGG (2021). Eetomgeving op scholen: Alles realistisch in beeld brengen. JOGG. (https://jogg.nl/nieuws/eetomgeving-op-scholen-alles-realistisch-in-beeld-brengen)

JOGG-aanpak (n.d.). JOGG. (https://jogg.nl/jogg-aanpak, 28 June 2021)

KFF (2021). Health Care Employment as a Percent of Total Employment. Kaiser Family Foundation. (https://www.kff.org/other/state-indicator/health-care-employment-as-total/)

Klause K (2018). Barcelona Superblocks: How Power and Politics Shape Transformational Adaptation. Barcelona Lab for Urban Environmental Justice and Sustainability. (http://www.bcnuej.org/2018/04/06/barcelona-superblocks-how-socio-political-power-struggles-shape-transformational-adaption/)

Kobes A, Kretschmer T, Timmerman MC (2021). Prevalence of overweight among Dutch primary school children living in JOGG and non-JOGG areas. PLoS One, 16(12):e0261406. (https://doi.org/10.1371/journal.pone.0261406)

Kochtitzky CS, Frumkin H, Rodriguez R et al. (2006). Urban Planning and Public Health at CDC (55(SUP02):34–38). (https://www.cdc.gov/mmwr/preview/mmwrhtml/su5502a12.htm)

Koeman J, Mehdipanah R (2021). Prescribing Housing: A Scoping Review of Health System Efforts to Address Housing as a Social Determinant of Health. Popul Health Manag, 24(3): 316–321. (https://doi.org/10.1089/pop.2020.0154)

Landes SD, Turk MA, Formica MK et al. (2020). COVID-19 outcomes among people with intellectual and developmental disability living in residential group homes in New York State. Disabil Health J, 13(4):100969. (https://doi.org/10.1016/j.dhjo.2020.100969)

Luxon L (2015). Infrastructure – the key to healthcare improvement. Future Hosp J, 2(1):4–7. (https://doi.org/10.7861/futurehosp.2-1-4)

Martínez A, Smith K, Llop-Gironés A et al. (2016). La mercantilización de la sanidad: El caso de Catalunya. Cuadernos de Relaciones Laborales, 34(2):335–355. (https://doi.org/10.5209/CRLA.53460)

Mehdipanah R, Rodríguez-Sanz M, Malmusi D et al. (2014). The effects of an urban renewal project on health and health inequalities: A quasi-experimental study in Barcelona. J Epidemiol Community Health, 68(9):811–817. (https://doi.org/10.1136/jech-2013-203434)

Mehdipanah R, Novoa AM, León-Gómez BB et al. (2019). Effects of Superblocks on health and health inequities: A proposed evaluation framework. J Epidemiol Community Health, 73(7):585–588. (https://doi.org/10.1136/jech-2018-211738)

Ministry of Health, Welfare and Sport (2019). The National Prevention Agreement [Rapport]. Ministerie van Algemene Zaken. (https://www.government.nl/documents/reports/2019/06/30/the-national-prevention-agreement)

Mueller N, Rojas-Rueda D, Khreis H et al. (2020). Changing the urban design of cities for health: The superblock model. Environ Int, 134:105132. (https://doi.org/10.1016/j.envint.2019.105132)

National Institute for Public Health and the Environment (2018). The Public Health Foresight Study 2018: A healthy prospect. National Institute for Public Health and the Environment. (https://www.vtv2018.nl/en)

National Institute for Public Health and the Environment (2020). Decrease in obesity in JOGG neighborhoods. (https://www.rivm.nl/nieuws/daling-overgewicht-in-jogg-buurten#%3A~%3Atext%3DIn%20buurten%20waar%20de%20JOGG%2Candere%20buurten%20zonder%20die%20aanpak)

Northridge ME, Freeman L (2011). Urban Planning and Health Equity. J Urban Health, 88(3):582–597. (https://doi.org/10.1007/s11524-011-9558-5)

Palència L, León-Gómez BB, Bartoll X et al. (2020). Study Protocol for the Evaluation of the Health Effects of Superblocks in Barcelona: The "Salut Als Carrers" (Health in the Streets) Project. Int J Environ ResmPublic Health, 17(8): 2956. (https://doi.org/10.3390/ijerph17082956)

Patil RR (2014). Urbanization as a determinant of health: A socioepidemiological perspective. Soc Work Public Health, 29(4):335–341. (https://doi.org/10.1080/19371918.2013.821360)

Pineda VS, Corburn J (2020). Disability, Urban Health Equity, and the Coronavirus Pandemic: Promoting Cities for All. J Urban Health, 97(3):336–341. (https://doi.org/10.1007/s11524-020-00437-7)

Quek Y-H, Tam WWS, Zhang MWB et al. (2017). Exploring the association between childhood and adolescent obesity and depression: A meta-analysis. Obes Rev, 18(7):742–754. (https://doi.org/10.1111/obr.12535)

Renders CM, Halberstadt J, Frenkel CS et al. (2010). Tackling the Problem of Overweight and Obesity: The Dutch Approach. Obes Facts, 3(4):267–272. (https://doi.org/10.1159/000319426)

Rico M, Font L, Arimon J et al. (2020). Informe qualitat de l'aire de Barcelona, 2020. Agència de Salut Pública de Barcelona. (https://www.aspb.cat/wp-content/uploads/2021/07/Informe_qualitat-aire-2020.pdf)

Ross CE, Mirowsky J (2001). Neighborhood Disadvantage, Disorder, and Health. J Health Soc Behav, 42(3):258–276. (https://doi.org/10.2307/3090214)

Rueda S (2016). La supermanzana, nueva celuca urbana para la construccion de un nuevo modelo funcional y urbanistico de Barcelona [The superblock, a new urban plan for the construction of a new functional and urban model for Barcelona]. (http://www.bcnecologia.net/es/proyectos/la-supermanzana-nueva-celula-urbana-para-la-construccion-de-un-nuevo-modelo-funcional-y)

Schwartz DF (2017). What You Need to Know About Hospital Roles in Community Investment. Culture of Health Blog. (http://www.rwjf.org/en/culture-of-health/2017/03/can-hospitals-defy-tradition.html)

Slot-Heijs J, Gutter K, Dellas V et al. (2020). Young people on a healthy weight in pictures 2015–2019 (p. 49). Mulier Institute. (https://www.mulierinstituut.nl/publicaties/25304/jongeren-op-gezond-gewicht-in-beeld-2015-2019/)

Sumah AM, Baatiema L, Abimbola S (2016). The impacts of decentralisation on health-related equity: A systematic review of the evidence. Health Policy (Amsterdam, Netherlands), 120(10):1183–1192. (https://doi.org/10.1016/j.healthpol.2016.09.003)

Taeuber KE, Taeuber AF (2009). Residential Segregation and Neighborhood Change. London: Routledge. (https://www.routledge.com/Residential-Segregation-and-Neighborhood-Change/Taeuber/p/book/9780202362793)

Tierney S, Wong G, Roberts N et al. (2020). Supporting social prescribing in primary care by linking people to local assets: A realist review. BMC Med, 18:49. (https://doi.org/10.1186/s12916-020-1510-7)

Torres ME (2019). Supermanzanas de Barcelona: El exitoso plan anticoches que arrancó con la oposición vecinal [Barcelona superblocks: the successful anti-car plan that started with neighbourhood opposition]. El País. (https://elpais.com/elpais/2019/10/07/icon_design/1570456123_584326.html)

Turk MA, Landes SD, Formica MK et al. (2020). Intellectual and developmental disability and COVID-19 case-fatality trends: TriNetX analysis. Disabil Health J, 13(3):100942. (https://doi.org/10.1016/j.dhjo.2020.100942)

United Nations (n.d.-a). Goal 11: Make cities inclusive, safe, resilient and sustainable. Sustainable Development Goals. (https://www.un.org/sustainabledevelopment/cities/, 28 June 2021)

United Nations (n.d.-b). Sustainable Cities and Communities—Make cities and human settlements inclusive, safe, resilient, and sustainable. (https://unstats.un.org/sdgs/report/2021/goal-11/, 8 September 2022)

United Nations Department of Economic and Social Affairs (2018). 68% of the world population projected to live in urban areas by 2050, says UN. (https://www.un.org/development/desa/en/news/population/2018-revision-of-world-urbanization-prospects.html)

United Nations Department of Economic and Social Affairs (n.d.). 11: Make cities and human settlements inclusive, safe, resilient and sustainable. (https://sdgs.un.org/goals/goal11, 28 June 2021)

WHO (1991). Technical Discussions on Strategies for Health for All in the Face of Rapid Urbanization: The Organization of Urban Health Systems (No. A44; pp. 1–19). World Health Organization. (https://apps.who.int/iris/bitstream/handle/10665/175459/WHA44_TD-4_eng.pdf?sequence=1&isAllowed=y)

WHO (2021). Global Health Workforce statistics database. (https://www.who.int/data/gho/data/themes/topics/health-workforce)

Zeng S, Pelzer KM, Gibbons RD et al. (2021). Consequences of COVID-19 vaccine allocation inequity in Chicago. medRxiv. (https://doi.org/10.1101/2021.09.22.21263984)

12 SDG13, *climate action: health systems as stakeholders and implementors in climate policy change*

IRIS A. HOLMES, CHARLEY E. WILLISON

12.1 Introduction

In August 2021 and March 2023, the Intergovernmental Panel on Climate Change (IPCC) starkly outlined humanity's inflection point with climate change: we must act now or face severe and irreversible consequences resulting from global warming driven by human emissions. Climate events directly threaten human health across a broad spectrum of issues – communicable diseases, heat events and natural disasters – which all present acute and chronic threats to human morbidity and mortality. Climate Action is one of the United Nation's Sustainable Development Goals. Yet despite calls for action, global governments have broadly not taken consequential change to reduce carbon outputs and mitigate warming. Our chapter argues that a primary cause of this inaction is political conflict and policy capacity. Without strong economic incentives and facing constrained resources, governments may opt to proceed with the status quo. Here, health systems present a critical resource to engage nations in climate action. Health systems produce political leverage as major political stakeholders across nations, globally, for *engaging* in broader climate policy and a wealth of resources inherent to health systems – expertise, funding – to directly *implement* climate policy.

The case study of the city of Toronto in Canada offers lessons for directly involving health systems in subnational climate action as policy stakeholders and implementors, and the co-benefits health system engagement brings to promote climate action intersectorally. Toronto provides an important case for high-latitude countries that will soon be facing climate hazards tropical nations have been grappling with for centuries. Engaging health systems in climate action policy processes may improve the likelihood of success for strengthening resilience and adaptivity to climate-related hazards.

12.2   What is SDG13 and how can health policy contribute?

Planetary health is inextricably related to human health. Anthropogenic climate change has been measurable since approximately 1900 CE (Crowley, 2000). The measurable effects of climate change increased substantially over the past two decades and will continue to accelerate in the future. We see these changes visibly in the increased frequency of natural and co-occurring natural and human-made disasters, adverse weather events including heat waves, sea level rise, and possibly the most salient, communicable disease transmission. The increase in individual events and their overlap necessitate immediate action to protect the health of the planet *and* the health of humans. This chapter outlines the unique position of health systems as 1) primary economic and political stakeholders in climate change policymaking and 2) essential actors in mitigating the adverse effects of climate change on human health. In both ways, health systems are vital actors in "strengthening resilience and adaptivity to climate related hazards and natural disasters" (SDG13 UN) related to anthropogenic climate change.

Health systems are primary parts of the economy and the political arena across all nations. In OECD nations, health accounts for a large part of government spending (OECD, 2019). While this amount varies across countries, health care systems across OECD countries account for a substantial proportion of social spending (OECD, 2019, 11). In some nations, health accounts for the greatest proportion of government spending on social programmes (for example, the United States). Spending on health systems in OECD nations will very likely increase in coming decades as population growth slows and citizens *age* substantially, necessitating increased health spending (OECD, 2021). Low-income countries will see increased need for spending on health systems as health risks increase with climate change (UNFCC, 2018).

While spending does not always translate directly to political engagement, health care sectors are major political stakeholders in OECD nations. High degrees of political leverage were engendered from long histories of policy engagement due to the professionalism of medicine and science (Best, 2019; Starr, 1982; Strach, 2015). Sustained political leverage for health systems also arises from the ways in which social policy systems have most often been structured around *health care*, as opposed to welfare, in OECD nations (Lynch & Perera, 2017; Starr, 1982; Tuohy, 2018). This centring of health care as opposed to social policy persists across OECD nations, even among lower-income OECD nations, where health systems may have sustained political leverage, even if publicly funded bureaucratic counterparts do not.

Health systems are also major contributors to climate change. For example, emissions from the US health care sector are among the highest (in absolute and per capita terms) of any health care system in the world, accounting for 8.5% of total greenhouse gas emissions nationwide in 2018 (Karliner et al., 2019; Medical Society Consortium on Climate and Health, 2021, 9; Pichler et al., 2019). Health care systems also exert substantial influence as consumers in general and are primary consumers for a number of specific industries. Examples include pharmaceutical manufacturing, which accounts for up to 10% of total greenhouse gas emissions in the United States (Belkhir & Elmeligi, 2019), and medical disposables (Campion et al., 2015), which can produce more carbon by up to a factor of ten than non-disposable alternatives (McGain et al., 2010; McPherson et al., 2019; Sherman et al., 2018). Per unit carbon emissions vary across pharmaceutical manufacturers (Belkhir & Elmeligi, 2019), implying that consumer choice by health care systems, or broad regulatory reforms, can lead to industry-wide improvements in emissions. In addition to consumption practices, simple, low-cost modifications to standard operating procedures can lead to significant energy and carbon savings. Surgical procedures in particular can be carbon intensive (MacNeill, Lillywhite & Brown, 2017). Much like pharmaceutical manufacturing, the carbon impact of different surgical approaches varies, implying potential for industry-wide improvement (Sherman et al., 2012).

Health systems can engage as leaders in reducing their outputs to mitigate climate change and have a direct interest in doing so to *reduce the adverse health effects of climate change*. Health systems around the globe will be a first line of defence for humans against the short- and long-term adverse health outcomes arising from climate change. Engaging health systems as key stakeholders in climate action policy processes upstream and downstream may improve the likelihood of success for strengthening resilience and adaptivity to climate-related hazards and natural disasters.

12.3   Causal pathways between health systems, climate change health action and co-benefits

Climate change is inextricably related to health outcomes. Health systems, as *upstream key stakeholders* in the political arena of most countries and *downstream responders*, or implementors to short- and long-term adverse health effects of climate change, are essential actors in achieving SDG13 climate change goals (see Fig. 12.1). The actions health systems take will likely produce co-benefits to other sectors through policy diffusion to produce intersectoral action in climate policy across other sectors, or direct climate mitigation benefits through internal health system changes.

12.3.1   *Responding to upstream climate change: health systems as critical economic and political stakeholders in driving support for climate change policy*

By virtue of the large proportion of political debates across OECD nations centred around health care and the economic prowess of health systems *themselves*, health systems are critical climate policy actors with the ability to shape agenda setting, influence political decisionmaking, and implement policies on the ground. Health systems can lead in climate policy debates and initiate policy change in other sectors and communities. Too long have health care and public health remained siloed from environmental health and climate concerns. Health systems are in a unique position to shift this notion and adopt a One-Health approach to climate action.

Many countries around the world are taking action to mitigate and prepare for climate change. Yet many more countries remain held back by various political factors contingent upon perceived benefits of engaging in climate change policy and institutional arrangements that may make policy action more or less viable. Agenda setting refers to whether or not topics become available to be considered for policy action (Kingdon, 1990; Schneider & Ingram, 1993; Stone, 1989). In countries where climate change is highly controversial, at the national or subnational level, *engaging health systems as critical political players* or stakeholders may improve the likelihood that climate policy is considered as a part of the political agenda in a jurisdiction (Stokes, 2020).

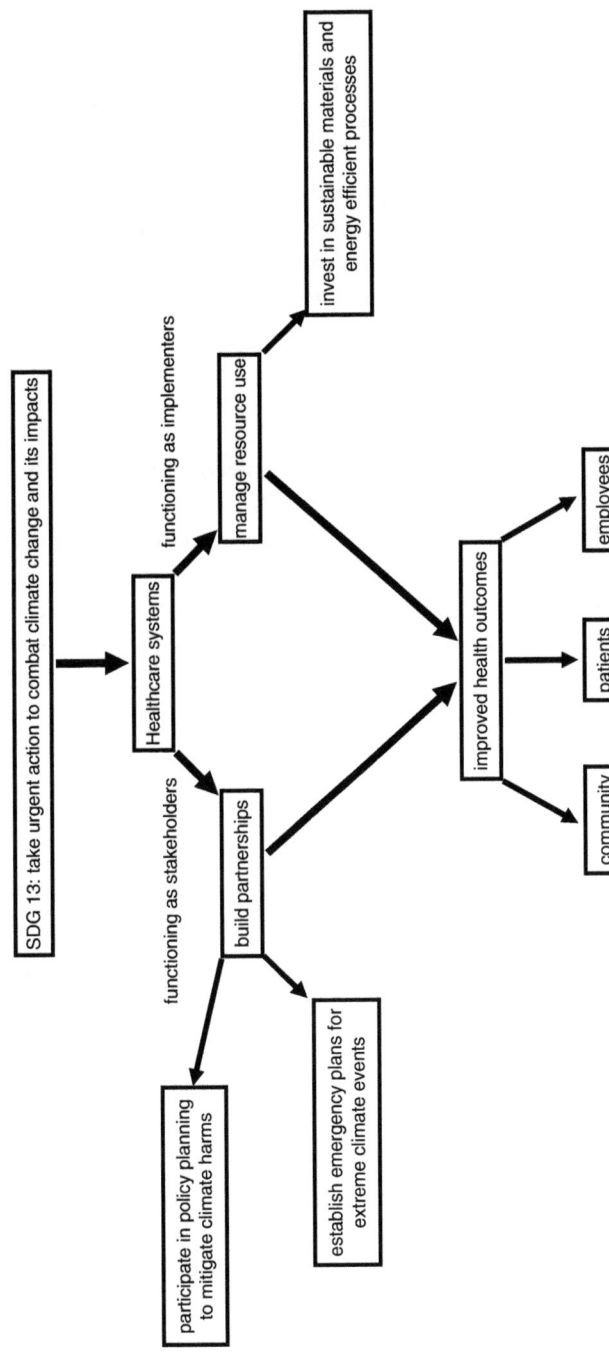

Fig. 12.1 Co-benefits for climate change through health system actions

Policy decisionmaking refers to the process by which political decisions are made that influence what policy outcomes, or formal or informal governmental actions on a specific topic, are generated or not. Policy decisionmaking is also influenced by a variety of complex factors. One critically important factor is the role of stakeholder groups. Stakeholder groups with stronger economic positions and coalitions of actors – large groups of well organized actors, such as professional organizations – wield more influence in political decisionmaking (Eaton & Weir, 2015). Health care systems across OECD nations persist as strong stakeholder coalitions because of their firm foothold in governmental spending valuing health care over other types of social policy, and economic power in privatized health systems (Beland & Waddan, 2012; Fox, 2016; Hacker et al., 2004; Kingdon, 1990; Starr, 1982; Tuohy, 2018). Once climate policy is on the agenda, organized mobilization by health systems may positively influence the likelihood of tipping national and subnational governments in favour of climate action, producing climate action co-benefits across jurisdictions.

Finally, health systems have crucial roles to play in policy implementation. Health system engagement in climate policy implementation may not only help speed implementation once policy has been generated but also help *initiate* policy action through diffusion. Policy diffusion is defined as occurring when one government's decision about whether to adopt a policy innovation is influenced by the choices made by other governments (Graham, Shipan & Volden, 2013, 675). Health systems, as key public or private stakeholders heavily involved in political decisionmaking across nations, have the ability to influence policy diffusion by acting as early adopters in climate change policy, while continuing to advocate for societal transition to renewable energy (Karliner et al., 2019, 36). Extensive co-benefits are produced when health systems engage in climate policy implementation across sectors, strengthening overall resilience and adaptivity (United Nations, 2021). Examples of climate policy implementation actions are outlined in the next section.

Policy diffusion is especially important in federated systems, where subnational governments may have varying degrees of adoption or movement towards climate policy. Yet policy diffusion can also happen intersectorally and internationally. Here, climate policy adaptation by health systems as primary components of a state may increase the likelihood of adoption of climate mitigation strategies by other state sectors (infrastructure, housing, education) or by other peer-countries (Bernauer,

2013, 437). There is much evidence to support policy diffusion as a mechanism for innovative or evidence-based health policies (Adolph et al., 2020; Grogan, Jones & Pacheco, 2017; Shipan & Volden, 2008; Tarr, 2001), and a growing body of evidence to support policy diffusion as a mechanism for environmental policies (Bromley-Trujillo et al., 2016). Health systems may help bridge the gap to facilitate policy diffusion across sectors. Health systems engaging in housing policy investments in the United States or lobbying for social spending in European nations (Lynch, 2019), are notable examples.

12.3.2   *Responding to downstream climate effects on health: health systems as essential actors in responding to and mitigating adverse effects of climate change in the short and long term*

The IPCC identifies major greenhouse gas emitting sectors as transport, buildings, industry, electricity, and land use practices, including agriculture and forestry. According to the COP21 glossary, decarbonization refers to the goal of energy-consuming processes producing no net (uncaptured) CO_2. As major consumers of energy and custodians of large building complexes, health care systems may be most directly positioned to influence those sectors toward decarbonization through the policy channels outlined above. In addition to upstream policy activities aimed at major and more formalized regulatory or legislative climate policy interventions, health care systems can act as policy implementors by taking immediate action within their own systems. Within-system changes may be particularly valuable in high-conflict contexts, which will be discussed shortly.

Downstream, direct actions taken by health care systems directly address a variety of climate-related health effects, while producing many intersectoral co-benefits. For example, health care systems can influence industry by setting low-carbon standards for their consumables, which account for 71% of the sector's emissions (Karliner et al., 2019, 5). Specific steps that health care systems could advocate for include investing in greener building materials for new construction or retrofitting old buildings to reduce carbon consumption for indoor climate control (Karliner et al., 2019). Additional benefits can be realized through investment in carbon-capturing green infrastructure, including living roofs and walls (Coutts & Hahn, 2015). Green buildings and open spaces provide important co-benefits particularly in the urban context, increasing the effectiveness and value of local ecosystem services such as runoff management (He et al., 2019) and capturing airborne particulate matter (Coutts & Hahn, 2015). Health outcomes and the importance of health care systems have historically been absent from the policy discussion around ecosystems services (Ford, Graham & White, 2015; Sandifer, Sutton-Grier & Ward, 2015). Health systems engaging in this area of policy could expand and improve the economic valuation of the quantifiable benefits (ecosystem services) provided by natural systems for human health as well as climate mitigation (de Groot et al., 2010; van Riper et al., 2017).

In addition to longer-term decarbonization investment, climate change is driving acute but unpredictable adverse events that are placing, and will continue to place, strong demands on health care systems. Health care systems are ideally situated to initiate or support policies designed to mitigate and manage the impacts of these events. Heat waves and emerging infectious diseases are classic examples of acute climate-driven hazards with unpredictable onset times that require management through policy. Natural disasters, such as hurricanes and wildfires, are described in more detail in the supplemental case study (Appendix 1). We describe the health threats posed by each category of event (heat waves and infectious diseases); discuss mitigation and planning strategies that would benefit from health system involvement; and demonstrate potential co-benefits emerging from action on these threats.

12.3.3   Heat waves

Climate change is predicted to drive longer, more intense, and more frequent heat waves, particularly in temperate regions that are not equipped to manage extreme heat (Arnell, Lowe & Challinor, 2019; Meehl & Tebaldi, 2004). Heat waves are defined as "a period of abnormally hot weather lasting longer than two days" by the United States National Weather Service. Heat waves increase morbidity and mortality, particularly in young children and the elderly (Haines et al., 2006; Herrmann & Sauerborn, 2018; Knowlton et al., 2009; O'Neill & Ebi, 2009). Exposure to chronic heat stress can lead to cardiovascular illness, chronic kidney disease, and mental health impacts (Kjellstrom et al., 2009; O'Neill & Ebi, 2009; Xiang et al., 2014). Manual labourers, including those who work outdoors such as farmers and construction workers, and those who may work with process-generated heat, such as factory workers and food service workers, are particularly at risk of negative impacts due to occupational exposure (Venugopal et al., 2020; Xiang et al., 2014).

12.3.4   Heat waves: the role of health systems and evidence-based actions

Health systems can work to mitigate the health impacts of heat waves in several specific ways. First, building green buildings and modifying open spaces to include tree cover can help mitigate the impacts of heat waves in buildings and in neighbouring areas, respectively (Aflaki et al., 2017; Onishi et al., 2010). In addition to saving cooling costs and the carbon emissions that come with air conditioning (Wong et al., 2003), these steps can help to buffer patients from indoor temperature swings, and will minimize impacts on particularly at-risk groups of employees such as food service workers and construction workers employed by health systems (Xiang et al., 2014). Higher vegetation cover at the neighbourhood scale (between 300m and 1km) can be correlated with improved health outcomes across a variety of measures, when neighbourhood and personal socioeconomic status are controlled for (Becker et al., 2019; Jenerette et al., 2016; Maas et al., 2009), indicating that investment in tree cover around health care facilities could benefit the surrounding neighbourhood as well as the specific buildings. Health systems can also participate in planning for heat waves. Many municipalities lack heat-wave response plans (Bernard & McGeehin, 2004). Health systems are well placed to raise awareness of the health impacts of heat waves, which may be less visible than those of other weather-related disasters. In addition, health systems have the expertise to help local governments develop plans for heat-wave response.

12.3.5   Emerging and migrating communicable diseases

Climate change is predicted to cause shifts in the ranges of many diseases currently restricted to warmer areas (Ciota & Keyel, 2019; Tesla et al., 2018) and to alter the relative prevalence and severity of pathogens throughout their ranges (Mordecai et al., 2020). High-latitude nations currently focused on chronic disease treatment will need to adapt their models of care to address emerging communicable diseases and should learn lessons from warm climate nations (Kavanagh & Singh, 2020).

Due to increasing temperatures, mosquito vectors of infectious disease are expanding their ranges toward the poles (Bartlow et al., 2019; Carvalho et al., 2015), as are parasites (York et al., 2015) and pathogens (Gonzalez et al., 2010; Maroli et al., 2008). From the perspective of any given location, the climate-driven shift in disease prevalence is unlikely to be predictable or orderly (Ciota & Keyel, 2019). At local levels, small differences in temperature microclimate can drive large differences in disease risk, particularly in vector-borne pathogens such as malaria, dengue or zika virus (Wimberly et al., 2020). Health systems will naturally be at the forefront of coping with emerging or migrating infectious diseases as they occur, but they can also play a role in preparing governments to cope with future threats.

12.3.6 Emerging and migrating communicable diseases: the role of health systems and evidence-based actions

Health systems can prepare for unpredictable and novel disease surges by planning for emerging epidemic diseases following procedures used to prepare for natural disasters. In addition to preparing for novel diseases, using green infrastructure in hospital grounds will reduce the local temperature and therefore the likelihood of an on-grounds disease outbreak. Incidence of viral diseases can track local temperature microclimates at the spatial scale of city blocks, with hotter neighbourhoods experiencing higher disease incidence (Wimberly et al., 2020), although socioeconomic status can be confounded with high local temperatures (Santos et al., 2020; Telle et al., 2021). Reducing local heat island effects could therefore mitigate the risk of a local outbreak.

Urban greening can also produce benefits for infectious disease management through a variety of mechanisms beyond reduction in local temperature. Vegetation increases surface permeability across cities, thereby slowing down runoff (He et al., 2019; Li et al., 2018; Mentens, Raes & Hermy, 2006). Slowing or reducing runoff volumes decreases the risk of runoff being contaminated with untreated sewage and other potentially dangerous substances (Zhang et al., 2015). Urban runoff often contains high concentrations of human-associated pathogens (Colford et al., 2012; Mallin & McIver, 2012), as well as pharmaceuticals, including antibiotics (Almakki et al., 2019). This combination can lead to the evolution of antibiotic resistance in potentially pathogenic bacteria strains (Almakki et al., 2019). Urban runoff can impact humans through direct contact and by contaminating agricultural systems and impacting food chains (Gillis, 2012). Health care buildings concentrate both pharmaceuticals and potential pathogens, making runoff management a high priority for the built environment of health care facilities (Devarajan et al., 2016; Kilunga et al., 2016; Laffite et al., 2016).

12.4 Governance and politics: conceptual issues

As discussed above, health systems bring an enormous amount of value to the table in their 1) upstream ability to promote climate change policy investments and 2) downstream, direct involvement in climate change mitigation through health and climate co-benefits, both short term and long term. Yet, while health systems have such substantial potential, the essential question persists: how do we attain these benefits? To answer this question, we must ask: 1) how do we actually *engage* health systems in climate change policy processes and 2) once health systems are on board, how do we mitigate conflict and constraints from other actors and systems to successfully promote climate change policy? To answer both questions, it is useful to think about: the degrees of conflict involved in climate policy discourse across governance systems; institutional constraints; and investments in health care systems.

Despite overwhelming and indisputable evidence of the reality of anthropogenic climate change from around the world, climate change is a policy space that still evokes high levels of *conflict* (see Table 12.1).

Table 12.1 *Health systems' potential to promote climate change policy*

| | | Conflict | |
		High	Low
Political importance	High	Health systems engage in bureaucratic decisionmaking, implementors in low-conflict jurisdictions	Health systems agenda setting, decisionmaking and implementation for policy diffusion
	Low	Health systems implementors in low-conflict jurisdictions	Health systems agenda setting, engage as implementors for policy diffusion

High levels of conflict arise in this policy space as a result of the threat (real and perceived) to existing economies and entrenched systems (Stokes, 2020; Stone, 1989). Thus, even when nations may place high degrees of political importance on addressing climate change, it may be met with substantial policy conflict arising from entrenched actors or coalitions, political parties, and the public (see Table 12.1) (Ansolabehere & Konisky, 2014; Peluso, Kearney & Lester, 2020). Coalitions and political parties centring opposition to climate policy starkly oppose climate interventions to protect status quo political economies they rely on (for example, fossil fuel industries and political parties with primary coalitions tied to these industries).

Institutional constraints interact with policy conflict. Institutional constraints refer to governance arrangements that make policy action more, or less, difficult at different levels (subnational vs. national) by placing different restrictions or checks on actors across multiple levels. Institutional constraints act as important accountability mechanisms and checks on power but may also inadvertently create barriers to policy action through fragmented systems and by gatekeeping political participation (see Tables 12.1 and 12.2). For example, highly fragmented and decentralized governance systems, such as in the United States, may necessitate more subnational action across policy mechanisms (agenda setting, decisionmaking and implementation) even in cases of high political importance and low policy conflict. Country context is very important in discerning institutional constraints that may impede or promote policy action and potential co-benefits (see Tables 12.1 and 12.2).

Table 12.2 *Potential to engage health systems in climate change policy*

		Stakeholder capacity	
		High	**Low**
Bureaucratic capacity	High	Health systems agenda setting, decisionmaking and implementation for policy diffusion	Health systems implementation for policy diffusion; localized or subnational decisionmaking
	Low	Health systems agenda setting	Health system engagement challenging

When seeking to engage health systems in climate change policy, the capacity of health systems and their capabilities or visibility as prominent stakeholders in a country context need to be considered (Gailmard & Patty, 2007). While health systems may be aware of the intractable relationships between climate change and health, both their bureaucratic and stakeholder capacity will likely determine health systems' ability to engage in policymaking and the potential for that engagement to be successful (see Table 12.2). Health systems' capacity or bureaucratic capacity refers to resource investments in health systems such as knowledge or expertise and resources to carry out expert recommendations (funding and staffing). For example, do health systems in a nation or jurisdiction have sufficient funding to make investments in decarbonization, ecosystem services, or disaster planning and mitigation?

Do health systems in a nation or jurisdiction have the expertise (internal and/or scientific and public health expertise through intersectoral co-benefits) to make systems investments through policy implementation or advocate on behalf of climate change policy through agenda setting and decisionmaking? Stakeholder capacity is related to bureaucratic capacity but refers to the degree to which health systems are considered prominent political actors or stakeholders in a country context. OECD nations, which invest substantial amounts of GDP in health systems, are likely to perceive health systems as high-capacity stakeholders, even if there is variation in subnational bureaucratic capacity of health systems (see Table 12.2). Low-income countries may see different arrangements regarding health system engagement in climate change policy dependent on policy context (see Table 12.2). For example, while having lower traditional measures of bureaucratic capacity for health systems in terms of spending and expertise, many low-income countries have very high levels of *bureaucratic expertise* in health systems specific to *infectious diseases*. Here, intersectoral action produces co-benefits between health systems' engagement with public health to generate high levels of policy mobilization in agenda setting and decisionmaking regarding communicable diseases and climate change, as seen in the COVID-19 pandemic (Kavanagh & Singh, 2020). Higher levels of bureaucratic capacity broadly or in specific policy spaces related to climate change, paired with higher levels of stakeholder capacity, may make health systems more likely to be engaged or become engaged in upstream climate change policy processes.

12.5   Case study: Toronto heat islands

12.5.1   *Toronto as a case of health system solutions to climate-exacerbated heat islands*

The case of solutions to climate-exacerbated urban heat islands (UHI) in the city of Toronto, Canada, acts as an exemplar case study of how health systems may act as policy implementors, driving action for policy diffusion in governmental climate debates. Toronto is a case of health systems policy engagement upstream *and* in policy implementation, producing co-benefits across sectors in climate change policy development.

Toronto is an ideal case for many reasons that may make it generalizable to other subnational and municipal governments around the globe. Toronto is a major, international city, comparable to other major metropolitan cities in OECD nations (City of Toronto, 2021). Major, global municipalities not only are primary *sites* of adverse effects of climate change including flooding and urban heat effects but also are experiencing increasing waves of growth and immigration. As major international city centres expand, municipalities like Toronto face domestic and international pressure to address these adverse effects, while also often having the ideology, wealth and intergovernmental transfers to do so (Sellers, 2002). Canada, like many OECD nations, is a Westminster system, with strong federated governance promulgating discretion in many policy spaces to subnational, here provincial, governments. In Canada, this federated arrangement plays a key role in the nation's national health system where the primary payer is the federal government, yet provinces have high degrees of autonomy on health care system delivery (Tuohy, 2018).

Heat islands are an ideal substantive policy case to examine the role of co-benefits because of their overlap in processes and outcomes related to health care systems, public health, ecosystems and disaster response. A set of mitigation strategies for Toronto's UHIs have now been in place for a decade or more, allowing comparisons between them and comparisons to the previous status quo. Modelling studies show that Toronto's ongoing mitigation strategies, including reflective pavement and building materials, green roofs and urban tree planting, can reduce mean temperatures in some areas by up to a degree during summer (Wang, Berardi & Akbari, 2016). This contribution improves human wellbeing directly and reduces energy demand on indoor climate control (Wang, Berardi & Akbari, 2016). These interventions reduce spending on energy, saving consumers up to $11 million CAD per year (Akbari & Konopacki, 2004). Such interventions are particularly critical, and particularly high-payoff, in areas zoned for commercial and industrial use (Rinner & Hussain, 2011; Wang, Berardi & Akbari, 2016). Heat waves in Toronto drive an approximate 10% increase in emergency services use over the baseline expectation, particularly in industrial areas (Dolney & Sheridan, 2006).

Increasing urban tree cover is correlated to measurable health benefits, significantly reducing the need for emergency care for heat-related morbidity during heat waves (Graham et al., 2016). Tree cover over 5% of ground surface was found to have a statistically significant association with heat-related health impacts in this study. By engaging in strategies such as urban greening and green roofs that both mitigate local health effects caused by the Toronto heat islands and capture carbon from the atmosphere, the Toronto approach furthers SDG13. Both the city's current efforts and the framework for future planning allow a proactive approach to reducing climate change and mitigating its ongoing impact. We investigate the development of UHIs to understand the role of health systems in upstream and downstream climate change policy processes, and the development of co-benefits produced from direct or indirect intersectoral engagement in these policy processes.

12.5.2 How SDG13 in Toronto produces co-benefits for other SDGs

Reducing climate change and mitigating its impact will further many of the UN's SDGs.[1] The case study of climate-related heat stress solutions in Toronto is an excellent example of these intersections. Climate

---

[1] By encouraging investment in greener technologies through their purchasing power, health systems can spur innovation and encourage scaling in clean energy, thereby forwarding SDG7. SDG8, decent work and economic growth, can be forwarded by the materials, labour and innovation necessary to retrofit health care infrastructure to reduce fuel waste or build new green infrastructure. Investment by such a large sector of the economy will provide jobs in the short term and build local skills for similar work throughout the economy. In addition, improving the physical environment within buildings will increase wellbeing among employees. Both through direct investment in sustainable buildings and through using their purchasing power to convince upstream industries to adopt greener manufacturing processes, health systems can impact SDG9, industry, innovation and infrastructure. Improvements in physical infrastructure and manufacturing processes driven by health system investment will spread to other, non-health-related, sectors of the economy. By more effectively managing their waste and investing in responsible waste-management

change-related droughts resulting from and exacerbated by heat effects are already limiting the availability of food and water to many vulnerable groups worldwide. SDG1, no poverty, and SDG2, zero hunger, are therefore made more challenging by climate change. SDG3, good health and wellbeing, is furthered by reducing heat stress within health system infrastructure and in surrounding areas. Evidence shows that reducing UHI effects and providing green spaces have broad impacts on health and wellbeing within local communities.

Many of the local climate mitigation strategies that health systems can engage in to reduce UHI, such as green infrastructure and urban greening, also reduce runoff and provide filtered urban water systems, contributing to SDG6, clean water and sanitation. Since health systems are major landowners within many cities, a pivot towards greener infrastructure can further SDG11, sustainable cities and communities. Health systems can participate in the political process of developing local or regional plans to mitigate and manage climate change, and can underline the urgency of such planning by providing evidence of ongoing climate-change-driven health impacts.

12.5.3 Policy timeline

Toronto was an early actor in North America and worldwide in preparedness for climate-exacerbated heat effects and in efforts to reduce and mitigate climate change. A series of policies enacted in Toronto, starting in 1999 (Clean Air Partnership, 2008), aimed at reducing climate change and mitigating adverse effects of climate change. For this case study we are focusing on *policies targeting UHIs* within the city, though there are many other climate policies in place. These policies targeting UHIs include: the Heat Health Alert System, a Green Roof Bylaw, the Toronto Green Standard, an Eco-Roof Incentive Programme, Doubling the Tree Canopy Initiative, and "Greening" Surface Parking Lot guidelines (Pacheco & Gower, 2016). Many of these policies relevant to UHI reductions have broader benefits to other categories of adverse climate

---

infrastructure, health systems can further SDG12, responsible consumption and production. Because of the necessity of single-use, sterile items in health care, health care systems generate large volumes of waste. Using their purchasing power to encourage sustainable and equitable waste management systems will reduce both the carbon footprint of health care and make waste management infrastructure available to other sectors.

events mitigation and preventing adverse health effects associated with climate change. We are focusing on the catalysing events for intersectoral policy action during the turn of the twenty-first century and will make comparisons across the past two decades to examine how Toronto has sustained these climate mitigation strategies to reduce UHIs.

12.5.4   Policy stakeholders

A key part of Toronto's success in early and sustained climate action is participation across a wide array of stakeholders relevant to heat stress mitigation. This stakeholder network includes actors involved in climate change mitigation strategies *and* those involved in responding to the downstream, adverse events arising from UHIs such as increased morbidity and mortality, adverse weather events, and infectious diseases (as outlined in Section 12.2). A key component of this process is that health systems were perceived to be both mitigators and responders to UHI climate events (Karliner et al., 2019). Health systems have also been involved as key stakeholders in these upstream and downstream roles in the policy process since 1999 and continue to be active today in climate policy agenda setting, decisionmaking and implementation. Toronto Public Health has also taken a direct role in all these policy activities since 1999, often leading policy decisionmaking and working to coordinate with health systems in their mitigation and response efforts (Acting Medical Officer of Health, 2016; Clean Air Partnership, 2008).

12.5.5   Co-benefits as an argument

In the policy discourse, co-benefits emerged in policy deliberations and rationale later on in the time period, appearing closer to 2020 (City of Toronto and Sustainability Solutions Group, 2019a). Co-benefits for climate resilience are now being adapted for measurable outcomes in the city of Toronto (City of Toronto and Sustainability Solutions Group, 2019b). While 'co-benefits' have not been consistently used until recently, Toronto's advocacy for intersectoral action and partnership across relevant actors in mitigation and response persisted across the two-decade time-period. Rationale for these intersectoral partnerships were based on the *benefits* to different actors and the necessity for partnerships to generate comprehensive and effective policy responses (Acting Medical Officer of Health, 2016; Health Canada, 2020). The recent emergence of co-benefits may be a product of the proliferation of this language by the UN, IPCC and other international climate change organizations.

12.5.6　Factors related to Toronto's success

Toronto's ability to lead as an early actor in various policies targeting UHIs is likely related to multiple political and governance factors. These factors are related to a *high level of intergovernmental and intersectoral collaboration*, and *high levels of policy capacity* to further these collaborations (see Table 12.3). High policy capacity in Toronto's case specifically included high capacity within the health system and the Toronto Department of Public Health to link health effects and target health outcomes to ecosystems services utilized to mitigate heat effects. Most important in many ways is the low level of political conflict and the high level of political support across levels and sectors of government (see Table 12.4). In these

Table 12.3 *Intersectoral governance structures in Toronto urban heat islands policies*

Tools			Possible governance actions with these tools								
			Goals and targets	Evidence support	Policy guidance	Implementation and management	Coordination	Advocacy	Monitoring and evaluation	Financial support	Legal mandate
Tools	Plan	Plan	X	X	X	X	X	X	X	X	X
	Indicators and targets	Indicators	X	X			X			X	
		Targets	X	X			X			X	
	Budgeting	Pooled budget									
		Shared objectives									
		Coordinated budgeting[2]	X							X	

[2]　Ontario Provincial Government (Acting Medical Officer of Health, 2016, 6).

Table 12.3 *(Cont.)*

			Possible governance actions with these tools						
Tools	Organization	Ministerial linkages[3]	X	X	X	X	X	X	X
		Specific ministers							
		Organization	X	X	X		X	X	
		Legislative committees							
		Interdepartmental committees/units	X	X	X		X	X	
		Departmental mergers							
		Civic engagement[4]	X	X	X	X	X	X	X
	Accountability	Transparent data							
		Regular reporting							
		Independent agency/ evaluators[5]	X	X	X	X	X	X	X
		Support for civil society[6]	X	X					
		Legal rights							

Table 12.4 *Political importance and conflict: the context of policymaking and implementation of Toronto urban heat islands policies*

		Conflict	
		Low	High
Political importance	High	x	
	Low		

[3] Toronto Environmental and Energy Departments (City of Toronto and Sustainability Solutions Group, 2019a, 26–28; Penney, 2012).
[4] Health Systems (Acting Medical Officer of Health, 2016).
[5] Canadian Federal Government (Health Canada, 2020; Toronto Medical Officer of Health, 2018).
[6] United Nations SDGs (Acting Medical Officer of Health, 2016, 10).

ways, Toronto's success may be relevant to other major metropolitan areas around the world. Major metropolitan areas, globally, tend to be more liberal and more progressive in climate policy action. In country contexts where either intersectoral or intergovernmental collaboration is missing or hindered, resulting from capacity or political conflict, health systems as major stakeholders may still be able to engage in action as implementors or spur action as agenda setters at the metropolitan level.

12.6   Discussion and conclusion

As key political stakeholders, health systems have the potential to promote substantial climate policy reforms. Health systems can take climate policy action to support SDG13 through upstream agenda-setting, and as directly implementing policy within their systems. We describe three categories of climate-driven, acute adverse events that are particularly amenable to mitigation through health system involvement: climate-driven natural disasters (discussed in the supplemental case study (Appendix 1)), communicable disease outbreaks, and heat waves. We conduct a case study analysis of the influence of health systems in climate policy development for responses to urban health islands (UHI) in Toronto, Canada. In Toronto, health system actors provided crucial policy capacity and stakeholder mobilization advocating for policy agenda-setting, policy design and implementation, while simultaneously producing policy co-benefits to other sectors through UHI mitigation.

Successful climate mitigation strategies will need to address governance challenges associated with political conflict and resource capacity, both upstream and downstream in policy design and implementation. Engaging health systems as primary economic stakeholders in national political economies may enhance the likelihood of climate policy success by generating upstream advocacy for climate policies and downstream capacity to implement policies on the ground. Toronto demonstrates this potential through intergovernmental health systems mobilization in response to UHIs. Even in cases where political conflict is high and capacity is low, health system climate policy action will produce cross-sectoral co-benefits arising from health systems as high-capacity implementors.

Health systems not only have capacity for policy change, but also have notable skin in the game as first-line responders to the adverse effects of climate change. Based on our findings from the analysis of co-benefits, governance challenges and Toronto as a case study, health systems as implementors may take immediate steps through both: 1) participating in local planning for adverse weather events, and 2) making direct infrastructure investments in sustainable buildings and materials. These actions will promote immediate progress for SDG13 and mitigate the health impacts of natural disasters, heat waves and emerging disease outbreaks.

References

Acting Medical Officer of Health (2016). Climate Change and Health Strategy: 2016 Update. (http://www.toronto.ca/legdocs/mmis/2014/hl/bgrd/backgroundfile-73622.pdf, 31 August 2021).

Adolph C, Amano K, Bang-Jensen B et al. (2020). Pandemic Politics: Timing State-Level Social Distancing Responses to COVID-19. medRxiv. (https://doi.org/10.1101/2020.03.30.20046326)

Aflaki A, Mirnezhad M, Ghaffarianhoseini A et al. (2017). Urban Heat Island Mitigation Strategies: A State-of-the-Art Review on Kuala Lumpur, Singapore and Hong Kong. Cities, 62(Feb):131–45. (https://doi.org/10.1016/J.CITIES.2016.09.003)

Akbari H, Konopacki S (2004). Energy Effects of Heat-Island Reduction Strategies in Toronto, Canada. Energy, 29(2):191–210. (https://doi.org/10.1016/J.ENERGY.2003.09.004)

Almakki A, Jumas-Bilak E, Marchandin H et al. (2019). Antibiotic Resistance in Urban Runoff. Sci Total Environ, 667:64–76. (https://doi.org/10.1016/J.SCITOTENV.2019.02.183)

Ansolabehere S, Konisky DM (2014). Cheap and Clean How Americans Think about Energy in the Age of Global Warming. Cambridge MA: MIT Press. (https://mitpress.mit.edu/books/cheap-and-clean)

Arnell NW, Lowe JA, Challinor AJ (2019). Global and Regional Impacts of Climate Change at Different Levels of Global Temperature Increase. Clim Change, 155(3):377–391. (https://doi.org/10.1007/S10584-019-02464-Z)

Bartlow AW et al. (2019). Forecasting zoonotic infectious disease response to climate change: mosquito vectors and a changing environment. Vet sci, 6(2):40.

Becker DA et al. (2019). Is green land cover associated with less health care spending? Promising findings from county-level Medicare spending in the continental United States. Urban For Urban Green, 41:39–47.

Béland D, Waddan A (2012). The politics of policy change: welfare, medicare, and social security reform in the United States. Georgetown University Press.

Belkhir L, Elmeligi A (2019). Carbon Footprint of the Global Pharmaceutical Industry and Relative Impact of Its Major Players. J Clean Prod, 214:185–194. (https://doi.org/10.1016/J.JCLEPRO.2018.11.204)

Bernard SM, McGeehin MA (2004). Municipal Heat Wave Response Plans. Am J Public Health, 94(9):1520. (https://doi.org/10.2105/AJPH.94.9.1520)

Bernauer T (2013). Climate Change Politics. Annu Rev Polit Sci. Annual Reviews. (https://doi.org/10.1146/annurev-polisci-062011-154926)

Best RK (2019). Common Enemies: Disease Campaigns in America. Oxford University Press.

Bromley-Trujillo R, Butler JS, Poe J et al. (2016). The Spreading of Innovation: State Adoptions of Energy and Climate Change Policy. Rev Policy Res, 33(5):544–565. (https://doi.org/10.1111/ropr.12189)

Campion N, Thiel CL, Woods NC et al. (2015). Sustainable Healthcare and Environmental Life-Cycle Impacts of Disposable Supplies: A Focus on Disposable Custom Packs. J Clean Prod, 94:46–55. (https://doi.org/10.1016/J.JCLEPRO.2015.01.076)

Carvalho BM et al. (2015). Ecological niche modelling predicts southward expansion of Lutzomyia (Nyssomyia) flaviscutellata (Diptera: Psychodidae: Phlebotominae), vector of Leishmania (Leishmania) amazonensis in South America, under climate change. PLoS One, 10(11):e0143282.

Ciota AT, Keyel AC (2019). The Role of Temperature in Transmission of Zoonotic Arboviruses. Viruses, 11(11). (https://doi.org/10.3390/V11111013)

City of Toronto and Sustainability Solutions Group (2019a). TransformTO: Climate Action for a Healthy, Equitable, Prosperous Toronto. (https://www.ssg.coop/transformto/, 24 September 2022)

City of Toronto and Sustainability Solutions Group (2019b). Benefits of Actions to Reduce Greenhouse Gas Emissions in Toronto: Climate Resilience. (https://www.toronto.ca/wp-content/uploads/2019/06/971c-Benefits-of-Actions-to-Reduce-Greenhouse-Gas-Emissions-in-Toronto-Climate-Resilience.pdf, 31 August 2021)

City of Toronto (2021). World Rankings for Toronto. Toronto's Dashboard. (https://www.toronto.ca/city-government/data-research-maps/toronto-progress-portal/world-rankings-for-toronto/)

Clean Air Partnership (2008). Climate Change Adaptation in the City of Toronto Lessons for Great Lakes Communities Clean Air Partnership. (https://glslcities.org/wp-content/uploads/2015/05/Toronto_ClimateChangeAdaptation.pdf)

Colford Jr JM et al. (2012). Using rapid indicators for Enterococcus to assess the risk of illness after exposure to urban runoff contaminated marine water. Water res, 46(7):2176–2186.

Counts NZ, Taylor LA, Willison CE, Galea S (2021). Healthcare Lobbying on Upstream Social Determinants of Health in the US. Prev med, 153.

Coutts C, Hahn M (2015). Green Infrastructure, Ecosystem Services, and Human Health. Int J Environ Res Public Health, 12(8):9768–9798. (https://doi.org/10.3390/IJERPH120809768)

Crowley TJ (2000). Causes of Climate Change Over the Past 1000 Years. Science, 289:5477. (https://science.sciencemag.org/content/289/5477/270/tab-pdf)

De Groot R et al. (2012). Integrating the ecological and economic dimensions in biodiversity and ecosystem service valuation. In Kumar P (ed.), The economics of ecosystems and biodiversity: Ecological and economic foundations (London: Routledge), 9–40.

Devarajan N, Laffite A, Kyela Mulaji C et al. (2016). Occurrence of Antibiotic Resistance Genes and Bacterial Markers in a Tropical River Receiving Hospital and Urban Wastewaters. PloS One, 11(2):e0149211. (https://doi.org/10.1371/JOURNAL.PONE.0149211)

Dolney T, Sheridan S (2006). The Relationship between Extreme Heat and Ambulance Response Calls for the City of Toronto, Ontario, Canada. Environ Res, 101(1):94–103. (https://doi.org/10.1016/J.ENVRES.2005.08.008)

Eaton C, Weir M (2015). The power of coalitions: advancing the public in California's public-private welfare state. Polit Soc, 43(1):3–32.

Ford AES, Graham H, White PCL (2015). Integrating Human and Ecosystem Health Through Ecosystem Services Frameworks. EcoHealth, 12(4):660–671. (https://doi.org/10.1007/S10393-015-1041-4)

Fox DM (2016). Health Policies, Health Politics. The British and American Experience, 1911–1965.

Gailmard S, Patty JW (2007). Slackers and Zealots: Civil Service, Policy Discretion, and Bureaucratic Expertise. Am J Pol Sci, 51(4):873–889. (http://www.jstor.org/stable/4620105)

Gillis PL (2012). Cumulative Impacts of Urban Runoff and Municipal Wastewater Effluents on Wild Freshwater Mussels (Lasmigona Costata). Sci Total Environ, 431:348–356. (https://doi.org/10.1016/J.SCITOTENV.2012.05.061)

González C et al. (2010). Climate change and risk of leishmaniasis in North America: predictions from ecological niche models of vector and reservoir species. PLoS Negl Trop Dis, 4(1):e585.

Graham DA, Vanos JK, Kenny NA et al. (2016). The Relationship between Neighbourhood Tree Canopy Cover and Heat-Related Ambulance Calls during Extreme Heat Events in Toronto, Canada. Urban For Urban Green, 20:180–186. (https://doi.org/10.1016/J.UFUG.2016.08.005)

Graham ER, Shipan CR, Volden C (2013). The Diffusion of Policy Diffusion Research in Political Science. Br J Polit Sci, 43(3):673–701. (https://doi.org/10.1017/S0007123412000415)

Grogan CM, Jones DK, Pacheco J (2017). Diffusion of ACA Policies across the American States. J Health Polit Policy Law, 42(2). (https://doi.org/10.1215/03616878-3766691)

Hacker JS et al. (2004). Privatizing Risk without Privatizing the Welfare State: The Hidden Politics of Social Policy Retrenchment in the United States. Am Polit Sci Rev, 98(2).

Haines A, Kovats RS, Campbell-Lendrum D et al. (2006). Climate Change and Human Health: Impacts, Vulnerability and Public Health. Public Health, 120(7):585–96. (https://doi.org/10.1016/J.PUHE.2006.01.002)

He Bao Jie, Jin Zhu, Dong Xue Zhao et al. (2019). Co-Benefits Approach: Opportunities for Implementing Sponge City and Urban Heat Island Mitigation. Land Use Policy, 86:147–157. (https://doi.org/10.1016/J.LANDUSEPOL.2019.05.003)

Health Canada (2020). Reducing Urban Heat Islands to Protect Health in Canada. (https://www.canada.ca/en/services/health/publications/healthy-living/reducing-urban-heat-islands-protect-health-canada.html, 31 August 2021).

Herrmann A, Sauerborn R (2018). General Practitioners' Perceptions of Heat Health Impacts on the Elderly in the Face of Climate Change—A Qualitative Study in Baden-Württemberg, Germany. Int J Environ Res Public Health 15(5). (https://doi.org/10.3390/IJERPH15050843)

Jenerette GD, Harlan SL, Buyantuev A et al. (2015). Micro-Scale Urban Surface Temperatures Are Related to Land-Cover Features and Residential Heat Related Health Impacts in Phoenix, AZ USA. Landsc Ecol, 31(4):745–760. (https://doi.org/10.1007/S10980-015-0284-3)

Jenerette GD et al. (2016). Micro-scale urban surface temperatures are related to land-cover features and residential heat related health impacts in Phoenix, AZ, USA. Landsc Ecol, 31:745–760.

Kaiser Permanente (2021). A Place to Call Home. Kaiser Permanente News. (https://about.kaiserpermanente.org/community-health/news/a-place-to-call-home, 16 January 2022)

Karliner J, Slotterback S, Boyd R et al. (2019). Health Care's Climate Footprint: How the Health Sector Contributes to the Global Climate Crisis and Opportunities for Action. (https://noharm-global.org/sites/default/files/documents-files/5961/HealthCaresClimateFootprint_092319.pdf)

Kavanagh MM, Singh R (2020). Democracy, Capacity, and Coercion in Pandemic Response: COVID-19 in Comparative Political Perspective. J Health Polit Policy Law, 45(6):997–1012. (https://doi.org/10.1215/03616878-8641530)

Kilunga PI, Kayembe JM, Laffite A et al. (2016). The Impact of Hospital and Urban Wastewaters on the Bacteriological Contamination of the Water

Resources in Kinshasa, Democratic Republic of Congo. J Environ Sci Health, 51(12):1034–1042. (https://doi.org/10.1080/10934529.2016.1198619)

Kingdon J (1990). Agendas, Alternatives and Public Policies. New York: Harper Collins.

Kjellstrom T, Butler AJ, Lucas RM et al. (2009). Public Health Impact of Global Heating Due to Climate Change: Potential Effects on Chronic Non-Communicable Diseases. Int J Public Health, 55(2):97–103. (https://doi.org/10.1007/S00038-009-0090-2)

Knowlton, K, Rotkin-Ellman M, King G et al. (2009). The 2006 California Heat Wave: Impacts on Hospitalizations and Emergency Department Visits. Environ Health Perspect, 117(1):61–67. (https://doi.org/10.1289/EHP.11594)

Laffite A, Kilunga PI, Kayembe JM et al. (2016). Hospital Effluents Are One of Several Sources of Metal, Antibiotic Resistance Genes, and Bacterial Markers Disseminated in Sub-Saharan Urban Rivers. Front Microbiol, 7:1128. (https://doi.org/10.3389/FMICB.2016.01128)

Li C, Liu M, Hu Y et al. (2018). Effects of Urbanization on Direct Runoff Characteristics in Urban Functional Zones. Sci Total Environ, 643:301–11. (https://doi.org/10.1016/J.SCITOTENV.2018.06.211)

Lynch J (2019). Populism, partisan convergence, and mobilization in Western Europe. Polity, 51(4):668–677.

Lynch JF, Perera IM (2017). Framing health equity: US health disparities in comparative perspective. J Health Polit Policy Law, 42(5):803–839.

Maas J et al. (2009). Morbidity is related to a green living environment. J Epidemiol Community Health, 63(12):967–973.

McGain F, McAlister S, McGavin A, Story D (2010). The financial and environmental costs of reusable and single-use plastic anaesthetic drug trays. Anaesth intensive care, 38(3):538–544.

MacNeill AJ, Lillywhite R, Brown CJ (2017). The Impact of Surgery on Global Climate: A Carbon Footprinting Study of Operating Theatres in Three Health Systems. Lancet Planet Health, 1(9):e381–388. (https://doi.org/10.1016/S2542-5196(17)30162-6)

McPherson B, Sharip M, Grimmond T (2019). The impact on life cycle carbon footprint of converting from disposable to reusable sharps containers in a large US hospital geographically distant from manufacturing and processing facilities. Peer J, 7:e6204.

Mallin MA, McIver MR (2012). Pollutant Impacts to Cape Hatteras National Seashore from Urban Runoff and Septic Leachate. Mar Pollut Bull, 64(7):1356–1366. (https://doi.org/10.1016/J.MARPOLBUL.2012.04.025)

Maroli M et al. (2008). The northward spread of leishmaniasis in Italy: evidence from retrospective and ongoing studies on the canine reservoir and phlebotomine vectors. Trop Med Int Health, 13(2):256–264.

Medical Society Consortium on Climate and Health (2021). The Costs of Inaction: The Economic Burden of Fossil Fuels and Climate Change on Health in the United States. (https://www.nrdc.org/sites/default/files/costs-inaction-burden-health-report.pdf)

Meehl GA, Tebaldi C (2004). More Intense, More Frequent, and Longer Lasting Heat Waves in the 21st Century. Science, 305(5686):994–997. (https://doi.org/10.1126/science.1098704)

Mentens J, Raes D, Hermy M (2006). Green Roofs as a Tool for Solving the Rainwater Runoff Problem in the Urbanized 21st Century? Landsc Urban Plan, 77(3):217–226. (https://doi.org/10.1016/J.LANDURBPLAN.2005.02.010)

Mordecai EA, Ryan SJ, Caldwell JM et al. (2020). Climate Change Could Shift Disease Burden from Malaria to Arboviruses in Africa. Lancet Planet Health, 4(9):e416–423. (https://doi.org/10.1016/S2542-5196(20)30178-9)

Muturi EJ, Alto BW (2011). Larval Environmental Temperature and Insecticide Exposure Alter Aedes Aegypti Competence for Arboviruses. Vector borne and zoonotic diseases (Larchmont, N.Y.), 11(8):1157–1163.

O'Neill MS, Ebi KL (2009). Temperature Extremes and Health: Impacts of Climate Variability and Change in the United States. J Occup Environ Med, 51(1):13–25. (https://doi.org/10.1097/JOM.0B013E318173E122)

OECD (2019). Health at a Glance 2019: OECD Indicators. Paris: OECD Publishing. (https://www.oecd-ilibrary.org/social-issues-migration-health/health-at-a-glance-2019_4dd50c09-en)

OECD (2021). Ageing and Long-Term Care – OECD. OECD. (https://www.oecd.org/els/health-systems/long-term-care.htm)

Onishi A, Cao X, Ito T et al. (2010). Evaluating the Potential for Urban Heat-Island Mitigation by Greening Parking Lots. Urban For Urban Green, 9(4):323–332. (https://doi.org/10.1016/J.UFUG.2010.06.002)

Pacheco E, Gower S (2016). Toronto's Heat Health Alert System Proactive Adaptation Can Help Save Lives Now and Prepare for Future Climate Change. (https://www.nrcan.gc.ca/changements-climatiques/impacts-adaptation/torontos-heat-health-alert-system/16295)

Peluso N, Kearney M, Lester R (2020). Assessing the Role of Public Policy in Industrial Transitions: How Distinct Regional Contexts Inform Comprehensive Planning. (https://ceepr.mit.edu/workingpaper/assessing-the-role-of-public-policy-in-industrial-transitions-how-distinct-regional-contexts-inform-comprehensive-planning/)

Pichler P-P, Jaccard IS, Weisz U et al. (2019). International Comparison of Health Care Carbon Footprints. Environ Res Lett, 14. (https://doi.org/10.1088/1748-9326/ab19e1)

Rinner C, Hussain M (2011). Toronto's Urban Heat Island—Exploring the Relationship between Land Use and Surface Temperature. Remote Sens, 3(6):1251–1265. (https://doi.org/10.3390/RS3061251)

Sandifer PA, Sutton-Grier AE, Ward BP (2015). Exploring Connections among Nature, Biodiversity, Ecosystem Services, and Human Health and Well-Being: Opportunities to Enhance Health and Biodiversity Conservation. Ecosyst Serv, 12:1–15. (https://doi.org/10.1016/J.ECOSER.2014.12.007)

Santos JPC et al. (2020). A perspective on inhabited urban space: land use and occupation, heat islands, and precarious urbanization as determinants of territorial receptivity to dengue in the city of Rio de Janeiro. Int J Environ Res Public Health, 17(18):6537.

Schneider A, Ingram H (1993). Social Construction of Target Populations: Implications for Politics and Policy. Am Polit Sci Rev, 87(2):334–347. (http://www.jstor.org/stable/2939044)

Sellers JM (2002). Governing from Below: Urban Regions and the Global Economy. Cambridge University Press.

Sherman JD, Raibley IV LA Eckelman MJ, (2018). Life cycle assessment and costing methods for device procurement: comparing reusable and single-use disposable laryngoscopes. Anesth Analg, 127(2):434–443.

Sherman J, Le C, Lamers V et al. (2012). Life Cycle Greenhouse Gas Emissions of Anesthetic Drugs. Anesth Analg, 114(5):1086–1090. (https://doi.org/10.1213/ANE.0B013E31824F6940)

Shipan CR, Volden C (2008). The Mechanisms of Policy Diffusion. Am J Polit Sci, 52(4). (https://www.jstor.org/stable/25193853?seq=1)

Starr P (1982). The Social Transformation of American Medicine. Basic Books.

Stokes LC (2020). Short circuiting policy: Interest groups and the battle over clean energy and climate policy in the American States. USA: Oxford University Press.

Stone DA (1989). Causal Stories and the Formation of Policy Agendas. Polit Sci Q, 104.

Strach P (2015). Hiding Politics in Plain Sight: Cause Marketing, Corporate Influence, and Breast Cancer Policymaking. New York: Oxford University Press.

Tarr GA (2001). Laboratories of Democracy? Brandeis, Federalism, and Scientific Management. Publius, 31(1):37–46. (https://doi.org/10.1093/oxfordjournals.pubjof.a004880)

Telle O et al. (2021). Social and environmental risk factors for dengue in Delhi city: A retrospective study. PLoS Negl Trop Dis, 15(2):e0009024.

Tesla B, Demakovsky LR, Mordecai EA et al. (2018). Temperature Drives Zika Virus Transmission: Evidence from Empirical and Mathematical Models. Proc Royal Soc B, 285:20180795. (https://doi.org/10.1098/RSPB.2018.0795)

Tuohy C (2018). Remaking Policy: Scale, Pace and Political Strategy in Health Care Reform. University of Toronto Press. (https://www.remakingpolicy.com/)

UNFCC (2018). Low-Income Countries Hit Hardest by Soaring Costs of Climate-Related Disasters. UNFCC News. (https://unfccc.int/news/low-income-countries-hit-hardest-by-soaring-costs-of-climate-related-disasters)

United Nations (2021). Goal 13 Climate Action: Take Urgent Action to Combat Climate Change and Its Impacts. Sustainable Development Goals. (https://www.un.org/sustainabledevelopment/climate-change/)

Van Riper CJ et al. (2017). Incorporating sociocultural phenomena into ecosystem-service valuation: the importance of critical pluralism. BioScience, 67(3):233–244.

Venugopal V, Latha PK, Shanmugam R et al. (2020). Occupational Heat Stress Induced Health Impacts: A Cross-Sectional Study from South Indian Working Population. Adv Clim Chang Res, 11(1):31–39. (https://doi.org/10.1016/J.ACCRE.2020.05.009)

Wang Y, Berardi U, Akbari H (2016). Comparing the Effects of Urban Heat Island Mitigation Strategies for Toronto, Canada. Energy Build, 114:2–19. (https://doi.org/10.1016/J.ENBUILD.2015.06.046)

Wimberly MC et al. (2020). Land cover affects microclimate and temperature suitability for arbovirus transmission in an urban landscape. PLoS Negl Trop Dis, 14(9):e0008614.

Wong NH, Cheong DKW, Yan H et al. (2003). The Effects of Rooftop Garden on Energy Consumption of a Commercial Building in Singapore. Energy Build, 35(4):353–364. (https://doi.org/10.1016/S0378-7788(02)00108-1)

Xiang J, Bi P, Pisaniello D et al. (2014). Health Impacts of Workplace Heat Exposure: An Epidemiological Review. Ind Health, 52(2):91–101. (https://doi.org/10.2486/INDHEALTH.2012-0145)

York EM et al. (2015). Geographic range expansion for rat lungworm in North America. Emerging Infect Dis, 21(7):1234.

Zhang Q, Miao L, Wang X et al. (2015). The Capacity of Greening Roof to Reduce Stormwater Runoff and Pollution. Landsc Urban Plan, 144:142–50. (https://doi.org/10.1016/J.LANDURBPLAN.2015.08.017)

Appendix
Case study: climate-driven health hazards – natural disasters

Natural Disasters

Climate change will continually increase natural disasters, particularly hurricanes and wildfires (Intergovernmental Panel on Climate Change, 2021; Shukla et al., 2019). Major disasters cause acute health impacts, notably from injury during flood-events (Blake & Zelinsky, 2017), and direct damage from smoke and particulate matter inhalation in the case of wildfires (Bowman & Johnston, 2005). Natural disasters also amplify infectious disease risk while simultaneously disrupting access to health services (Sharma et al., 2008; Willison & Holmes, 2020). When disasters force people from their homes, they often gather in congregate facilities. Group housing presents high-risks for contagious diseases, such as influenza or noroviruses (Loebach & Korinek, 2019). Hurricanes and flood-related disasters provide ideal breeding situations for arthropod-disease-vectors, causing outbreaks in the weeks and months following the disaster (Beatty et al., 2007). Finally, disaster events can cause or exacerbate chronic health conditions. Notably, particulate matter from fires can increase chronic respiratory and cardiovascular disease (Liu et al., 2015). Hurricanes and flood-events account for direct, indirect, acute and chronic adverse health effects primarily related to: behavioural health challenges, socioeconomic loss, infrastructure damage (mould, housing loss), and contamination from pollutants during storm surges (Waddell et al., 2021).

Natural disasters: the role of health systems and evidence-based actions

Health systems can act as policy implementors by investing in green buildings and greening open spaces in health care infrastructure, mitigating the acute impacts of climate-driven natural disasters. Urban greening, particularly with broadleaf trees, can reduce particulate-matter-density in the air (Deng et al., 2019; Lei et al., 2021) exacerbated during climate-driven disasters including heat waves and wildfires. Urban greening also increases surface permeability, slowing down runoff during flood-related disasters and reducing risk of contamination with sewage or other dangerous substances (He et al., 2019; Li et al., 2018).

References

Beatty ME et al. (2007). Mosquitoborne Infections after Hurricane Jeanne, Haiti, 2004. Emerging Infect Dis, 13(2):308. (https://doi.org/10.3201/EID1302.061132)

Blake ES, Zelinsky DA (2017). National Hurricane Center Tropical Cyclone Report: Hurricane Harvey. (https://www.nhc.noaa.gov/data/tcr/AL092017_Harvey.pdf)

Bowman D, Johnston F (2005). Wildfire Smoke, Fire Management, and Human Health. *EcoHealth* 1(2). (https://researchers.cdu.edu.au/en/publications/wildfire-smoke-fire-management-and-human-health)

Deng T et al. (2019). Shrinking cities in growing China: Did high speed rail further aggravate urban shrinkage? Cities, 86:210–219.

He D et al. (2022). Urban greenery mitigates the negative effect of urban density on older adults' life satisfaction: Evidence from Shanghai, China. Cities, 124:103607.

Intergovernmental Panel on Climate Change (2021). Summary for Policymakers. In Masson-Delmotte et al. (eds), Climate Change 2021: The Physical Science Basis. Contribution of Working Group I to the Sixth Assessment Report of the Intergovernmental Panel on Climate Change (Cambridge University Press).

Lei Y et al. (2021). Scale-dependent effects of urban greenspace on particulate matter air pollution. Urban For Urban Green, 61:127089.

Li J et al. (2020). An evaluation of urban green space in Shanghai, China, using eye tracking. Urban For Urban Green, 56:126903.

Liu JC, Pereira G, Uhl SA et al. (2015). A Systematic Review of the Physical Health Impacts from Non-Occupational Exposure to Wildfire Smoke. Environ Res, 136(January):120–132. (https://doi.org/10.1016/J.ENVRES.2014.10.015)

Loebach P, Korinek K (2019). Disaster Vulnerability, Displacement, and Infectious Disease: Nicaragua and Hurricane Mitch. Popul Environ, 40(4):434–455. (https://doi.org/10.1007/S11111-019-00319-4)

Sharma AJ et al. (2008). Chronic Disease and Related Conditions at Emergency Treatment Facilities in the New Orleans Area after Hurricane Katrina. Disaster Med Public Health Prep, 2(1):27–32. (https://doi.org/10.1097/DMP.0B013E31816452F0)

Shukla PR et al. (2019). Technical Summary, 2019. In Climate Change and Land: An IPCC Special Report on Climate Change, Desertification, Land Degradation, Sustainable Land Management, Food Security, and Greenhouse Gas Fluxes in Terrestrial Ecosystems (United Nations: Intergovernmental Panel on Climate Change). (https://www.ipcc.ch/site/assets/uploads/sites/4/2019/11/03_Technical-Summary-TS.pdf)

Waddell SL, Jayaweera DT, Mirsaeidi M et al. (2021). Perspectives on the Health Effects of Hurricanes: A Review and Challenges. Int J Environ Res Public Health, 18(5):2756. (https://doi.org/10.3390/IJERPH18052756)

Willison C, Holmes I (2020). Isolated Coronavirus Policies and Models Create Perverse Incentives for Disaster Preparedness. (https://doi.org/10.1599/mqop.2020.0730)

13 SDG17, *means of implementation: strengthen the means of implementation and revitalize the Global Partnership for Sustainable Development*

HOLLY JARMAN

13.1 Introduction

Sustainable Development Goal 17, to 'strengthen the means of implementation and revitalize the Global Partnership for Sustainable Development' (United Nations, 2022) is a little different from some of the other goals covered in this book. At first glance, you would be forgiven for thinking that SDG17 is a 'grab bag' of aspirations; that it covers everything not covered by the other goals. Its scope is very broad, covering finance, taxation, debt and capital flows, governance and multi-stakeholder partnerships, international trade and aid, technology diffusion, shared knowledge, shared data, capacity building and national planning (United Nations, 2022). SDG17 has a history of conceptual slipperiness, and even its fundamental definition can change in different contexts. Some sources emphasize SDG17's reference to the "means of implementation" foregrounding the financial and technical capabilities seen as necessary to achieve sustainable development (Eurostat, 2022; United Nations, 2018). Others elaborate on the theme of partnership and translate this into literal multi-stakeholder partnerships for facilitating or renewing sustainable development (Addo-Atuah et al., 2020; Leal Filho, 2022; Oliveira-Duarte et al., 2021).

What is strange in terms of policymaking is that it is rare to find so many big, important policy areas addressed in one policy framework. Where the norm in policymaking is most often to have a strong segregation between "core" (often economic) policy areas and aspects of social and environmental policy, SDG17 has the potential to force governments, including health ministries, to consider how these policy areas interact and influence one another. From this standpoint, SDG17 is a potentially great

250

framework to consider co-benefits, the intersectoral positive spillovers between health and other policy areas. It can be viewed as a means of facilitating some of the cooperation across policy areas that we are told is much needed (see Chapters 1–4 of this volume; Greer et al., 2022a), and of better understanding (and even mitigating) negative intersectoral spillovers.

But also because of its breadth, SDG17 might be one of the most ambitious SDGs. In order to make progress towards SDG17, states need to work together to create more equitable systems for trade, aid, debt and knowledge sharing at the global level as well as improve the governance and administrative capacity of individual states and their relationships with third party stakeholders and civil society groups. This is a tall order. There could be a significant risk that SDG17, defined too concretely, might not be achieved on any reasonable timeframe, or at all. SDG17 balances out its ambition by keeping its goals vague, aspirational and sometimes hard to measure. In terms of allowing countries to work together over the longer term, this could be an advantage. Each can claim progress without seeming to have "failed" to reach certain benchmarks or milestones. That flexibility can enable promises but leaves the risk of delivering very little, with no ability for third parties to hold governments to account when they fail to deliver on their promises.

This chapter examines the wide-ranging and often poorly defined SDG17 in the context of health policy and governance. Health policies and systems, including public health policies, as well as the general state of population health, affect the key components of SDG17 in important ways, from facilitating trade and economic growth to using the power of health care systems as large purchasers and employers. How can health policies and systems provide co-benefits that contribute to achieving goals from SDG17?

I argue that there are significant synergies between health policy and SDG17. Many of the factors that potentially make "sustainable development" possible require healthy populations and functional health systems. Just as factors like trade and capital flows, good enough governance, a clean environment, or access to technology are very important determinants of health, good population health and the systems that make that possible are essential for achieving sustainable development. The COVID-19 pandemic has made these synergies very visible across the world, in terms of both the importance of international cooperation as well as the consequences of its failure. I argue that none of the potential co-benefits can be achieved without health actors at the table, as the pandemic makes clear. The next sections examine the content of SDG17 and explore the co-benefits with health, before placing the framework in the context of the COVID-19 pandemic.

13.2   What does SDG17 cover? What are the co-benefits between these areas and health?

SDG17 covers a lot of ground and might seem confusing (see Table 13.1), but it is actually a very strong embodiment of the key tenets of "sustainable development" (Sachs, 2015). On the one hand, its core priorities are mostly economic, including trade, investment, capital flows, aid and debt relief. But while the SDG promotes and centres economic growth, it does not promote just any growth. In each of these areas of economic policy, consideration is given to how a mixture of multilateral cooperation and enhancing national capacity can create more stable growth over time that is more equally distributed among states. In order to further these goals, SDG17 includes a range of areas that could be considered technical improvements to existing systems, such as improving technology

Table 13.1 *The main elements of SDG17*

Element	Policies
Finance and aid	Overseas development assistance
	Foreign direct investment (and investment promotion schemes)
	Remittances
	Debt financing, relief and restructuring
	Government revenue and ability to collect taxes
	Maintain stable macroeconomic climate, e.g., reduce boom and bust, rapid capital flows
Trade	Promote a "universal, rules-based, open, non-discriminatory and equitable multilateral trading system"
	Significantly increase exports of developing countries
	Reduce tariffs for developing countries, Least Developed Countries and small island states

Table 13.1 *(Cont.)*

Element	Policies
Governance, capacity building and multi-stakeholder partnerships	Technical and financial assistance
	"Enhance policy coherence of sustainable development"
	Respect each country's policy space and leadership to establish and implement policies for poverty eradication and sustainable development
	Promote multi-stakeholder partnerships
	Enhance the global partnership for sustainable development, complemented by multi-stakeholder partnerships that mobilize and share knowledge, expertise, technology and financial resources, to support the achievement of the Sustainable Development Goals in all countries, in particular developing countries
	Promote effective public–private and civil society partnerships
Access to science, technology and innovation	Internet and broadband access
	Knowledge sharing agreements
	Improve access to environmentally sound technologies, e.g., via technology transfer
Data	Enhance statistical capacity, create national statistical plans, improve birth and death records
	By 2030, build on existing initiatives to develop measurements of progress on sustainable development that complement gross domestic product, and support statistical capacity-building in developing countries

transfer and dissemination of scientific knowledge in ways that can foster growth. Improving government capacity to govern is also addressed, for example, a state's ability to keep records, share data or collect taxes.

As such, the main critiques of SDG17 are those that apply to the concept of sustainable development itself – the objectives outlined by SDG17 are more often about "greening" the global economic system or redistributing its benefits rather than reconstituting the system in any significant way (Lafferty, 1996; Mitlin, 1992; Weber & Weber,

2020). While sharing the benefits of growth more equally among states is a key goal, SDG17 does not explicitly centre equity and focuses on differences between countries rather than inter-population disparities. From this perspective, SDG17 is more about politics than power. States aspire to "respect each country's policy space and leadership" (Target 15) and promote "multi-stakeholder partnerships that mobilize and share knowledge" (Target 16) rather than reform the ways that governments vote or create multilateral institutions focused on massive wealth redistribution, for example.

The objectives in SDG17 and their associated measurements can seem vague and incoherent – one of the targets is itself to "enhance policy coherence of sustainable development" (Target 14), measured by the "number of countries with mechanisms in place to enhance policy coherence of sustainable development". Nevertheless, examining the key themes within SDG17 collectively makes clear their importance to each other, and the importance of health policies, health care and the health system to them.

For anyone who pays attention to population health, one ongoing frustration stems from the fact that many aspects of health are determined by policies and systems outside the health domain (Evans, Barer & Marmor, 1994; Marmot & Allen, 2014). That explains why there is an extensive literature on the ways in which elements of SDG17 such as trade policy affect health systems and outcomes. To be healthy, people need access to adequate amounts of healthy, sustainable and culturally appropriate food, for example. While mass manufacturing and liberalized trade can increase food availability, it is not guaranteed that the new food will be nutritious, produced in environmentally sound ways, or a good fit with local ways of eating and procuring food. Changes in trade patterns on Pacific islands leading to an influx of cheap, high-calorie food and related advertising have been shown to impact local diets in negative ways (Friel et al., 2013; Hughes & Lawrence, 2005; MacKenzie & Collin, 2012; Snowdon & Thow, 2013; Thow et al., 2010). Furthermore, market liberalization can create an influx of, and demand for, new, unhealthy goods such as tobacco products and undermine related public health policies in important ways (Crosbie et al., 2021; Drope & Lencucha, 2013; Jarman, 2015, 2019; Lee et al., 2009; McGrady, 2011; Shaffer, Brenner & Houston, 2005). In addition to impacting the flow of goods, changes in trade can also structure employment opportunities and related population flows in ways that shape working environments, living conditions and social structures. While work can be vital to live, the nature of work affects quality of life in significant ways. Increasing the volume of trade does not guarantee equitable distribution of its profits and may increase inequities over time. Good population health thus relies not just on economic growth but also on how the benefits of growth are distributed (Marmot et al., 2010, 2020; WHO Commission on Social Determinants of Health, 2008).

Understanding the inverse relationship – the impact of health on SDG17 – is equally important (Table 13.2). Achieving any measure of global economic equity without progress in global health equity seems unlikely. Populations in poor health – with either higher mortality rates and/or higher morbidity – cannot contribute as much towards the global economy in terms of labour, productivity and innovation. The global burden of communicable and non-communicable disease is a barrier to sustainable growth, as are barriers to accessing needed health care, whether preventative, routine or urgent (GBD 2019, 2020). States do not create and maintain health systems purely out of altruism or a sense of upholding rights to health, although this may be part of their justification. Adequate health care that is accessible at the point of need and not unduly costly or burdensome is a key component of a successful economy. So, too, are the public health structures that detect, and aim to prevent, the spread of communicable disease (Acemoglu & Johnson, 2007; Alkire et al., 2018; GBD, 2020; Remes et al., 2020; Sharma, 2018).

Good population health and health care access support the global economy. But the health sector itself can also be a source of economic benefits and employment. In many countries, the health sector provides a significant number of jobs, fosters new research and disseminates scientific knowledge. Health sectors in EU countries, for example, have been shown to produce high added value and significant employment, despite being relatively independent of other sectors in the economy (Gutiérrez-Hernández & Abásolo-Alessón, 2021). In addition, most health organizations, both those funded by governments and those funded by private spending, exist as part of services and goods trade within the global economy. In 2019, prior to the COVID-19 pandemic, the top five exporting countries in pharmaceuticals accounted for $319.68 billion in exports, while the top five countries exporting medical devices accounted for $126.71 billion (Skrzypek, 2020). In terms of trade in services, WHO projects that increased health care demand will

Table 13.2 *Potential co-benefits from good population health and the health sector for achieving SDG17*

Element	Population health potential co-benefits	Health sector potential co-benefits
Finance and aid Overseas development assistance; foreign direct investment (and investment promotion schemes); remittances; debt financing, relief, and restructuring; government revenue and ability to collect taxes; maintain stable macroeconomic climate, e.g., reduce boom and bust, rapid capital flows	• Facilitates workforce participation and productivity, supporting overall economic growth and government revenue • Physically and mentally healthy workforce and absence of communicable diseases in the population provide value to businesses and investors • Investment and aid are more likely to result in growth when population is healthy	• Prevention of communicable disease spread, e.g., vaccination, can support economic stability • Fewer disruptions to economic activity, greater productivity when workforce can access health care • Businesses benefit from collectively funded and managed health systems
Trade Promote a "universal, rules-based, open, non-discriminatory and equitable multilateral trading system"; significantly increase exports of developing countries; reduce tariffs for developing countries, Least Developed Countries and small island states	• A healthy workforce is an essential part of the infrastructure required to trade successfully • Controlling communicable disease outbreaks prevents supply chain disruptions	• Trade in health services can be a source of economic growth • Can be a source of profitable exports, e.g., trade in pharmaceuticals and medical devices

Governance, capacity building and multi-stakeholder partnerships Technical and financial assistance; "Enhance policy coherence of sustainable development"; respect each country's policy space and leadership; promote multi-stakeholder partnerships; enhance the global partnership for sustainable development, complemented by multi-stakeholder partnerships	• Healthy population facilitates civic engagement and multi-stakeholder partnerships • A healthier population is better able to hold policy decisionmakers and political leaders to account • Healthier populations may be better able to participate in global partnerships and policy spaces • Healthier populations may be better able to take advantage of technical and financial assistance	• Health sector contains many examples of successful multi-stakeholder partnerships • Health systems are key partners in progress towards sustainable development
Access to science, technology and innovation Internet and broadband access; knowledge sharing agreements; improve access to environmentally sound technologies, e.g., via technology transfer	• Healthy people may have more ability to engage in education and training	• Fosters new research, disseminates scientific knowledge • Innovation in new health products and services supports economic growth and innovation in other sectors

Table 13.2 (*Cont.*)

Element	Population health potential co-benefits	Health sector potential co-benefits
Data Enhance statistical capacity, create national statistical plans, improve birth and death records; by 2030, build on existing initiatives to develop measurements of progress on sustainable development that complement gross domestic product, and support statistical capacity-building in developing countries	• A healthy population supports statistical and analytic capacity within a country	• Health sector is a source of expertise on population statistics and analysis • Health sector generates data of value to governments, businesses, researchers and civil society (see Chapter 9)

result in 84 million health care jobs, mostly in high- and middle-income countries, by 2030 – a 29% growth rate (Boniol et al., 2022). This is a demand rich countries will try to meet with a combination of domestic investment and foreign recruitment, including international medical education (for example, French students studying medicine in Romania or German students studying dentistry in Austria). Across eight European countries in a recent study, the number of foreign-trained doctors increased by over 46% between 2010 and 2018 (Williams et al., 2020).

Overall, these examples show how interconnected population health, health care and the global economy really are, but they also point to the challenges that this poses for sustainable development. For example, is increased health care professional mobility a good thing? Recruitment of foreign health care workers can help to meet workforce needs in high-income countries but may cause "brain drain" in countries with limited capacity to train new doctors and nurses (Wismar et al., 2011). As commercial actors, pharmaceutical companies can create big profits and support growth and innovation, but the products they create may not match the need for more basic medicines and may not be accessible for poorer countries due to cost and strong intellectual property pro-tections that limit the production of generic medicines. What happens to health markets when governments spending a significant proportion of GDP on health care come under pressure to reduce spending and government debt? Or to our understanding of contemporary health problems when commercial actors collect and maintain more relevant health data than governments? Is it possible within the constraints of this SDG to improve equity within national borders?

As such, the co-benefits between SDG17 and health may not be attained without integrating people who understand health care and the drivers of population health into spaces designed for economic policymaking (Jarman & Koivusalo, 2017; Koivusalo, 2014). But the process for making decisions on economic issues including taxation, industrial policy, trade, debt, investment or intellectual property is frequently divorced from the governance of health policy (Jarman, 2017). A degree of alignment and common discourse between actors responsible for the economic components of SDG17 and health policy stakeholders is likely needed to achieve meaningful progress.

In the text of SDG17, much of the weight of this integration is carried by the concept of a "multistakeholder partnership", driven by the central assumptions that 1) bringing organizations from multiple sectors and perspectives into dialogue will create "policy coherence" across issue boundaries and 2) effective policy implementation requires the knowledge, data and financial resources of actors outside the realm of government. As such, the concept is part of an intellectual framing that has long been part of how the WHO operates (Yamey, 2002).

Decisions about forming partnerships need to be handled carefully. Studies of the commercial determinants of health show that while bringing in actors with vested interests might potentially make policies more coherent, companies with vested interests tend to push policy debates towards ineffective or weak solutions such as industry self-regulation (for a summary, see Maani et al., 2020; Maani, Petticrew & Galea, 2022). Companies, by definition, are designed to support the interests of their shareholders over the concerns of health advocates, and a range of firms producing products such as tobacco, alcohol, food, pharmaceuticals and cars have had damaging effects on policies meant to protect health.

Nevertheless, having health actors, particularly public health actors, engaged in multi-stakeholder partnerships is essential for meeting the goals of SDG17; they can do much more than just block bad policy ideas. Health partners can promote policy coherence in service of sustainable development by bringing an understanding of how human health facilitates or puts at risk sustainable growth, an appreciation of the cross-border nature of many of these determining factors, a range of robust methods for collecting and disseminating comparable and reliable data, and a longstanding body of evidence supporting preventative actions to improve health before problems develop.

The next section explores this question of alignment in the context of the ongoing COVID-19 pandemic, with specific focus on sustainable food systems, collaboration to develop and distribute vaccines, and the collection and sharing of relevant health data.

13.3   How have we performed on SDG17 during the COVID-19 pandemic?

The COVID-19 pandemic has shown us just how much the connections between sustainable development and health matter, but also, unfortunately, how weak global cooperation can be during a crisis. Health policies adopted as responses to the COVID-19 pandemic have impacted performance across all areas of SDG17 (see Table 13.3). Although many in the international community have called for "global solidarity" in

Table 13.3 *Elements of SDG17 in the context of the COVID-19 pandemic*

Element	Importance of SDG element to pandemic response	Health sector importance to SDG element	Impacts of pandemic response on SDG element
Finance and aid	Required by low resource countries to buy medicines/equipment and for staffing; required to keep populations healthy during economic downturn; required to prevent widening inequality	Healthy populations support stable financial systems; health sectors support related growth and can provide revenue	Pandemic response impacts economic stability and performance, which can affect governments' and investors' ability or will to provide finance/aid or individuals' ability to send home remittances; travel bans, supply chain disruptions and lockdowns may impact ability to disperse aid; focus on pandemic-related aid/finance may reduce pressure to provide routine aid/finance
Trade	Allows distribution of treatments and vaccines; vital for distribution of food and other immediate needs; supports economic growth and recovery	Healthy populations support growth in trade volumes; health systems can contribute to trade in services; the health sector is a source of innovative products for export	The extent to which a government takes action to curb disease outbreaks, its choice of policy actions and its support for the population through social policies has multiple cross-cutting effects on trade volumes and supply chain resilience, e.g., impacting domestic production for export, availability of imports, stability of global markets

Table 13.3 (Cont.)

Element	Importance of SDG element to pandemic response	Health sector importance to SDG element	Impacts of pandemic response on SDG element
Governance, capacity building and multi-stakeholder partnerships	Support procurement and distribution of treatments and vaccines, contact tracing capacity, testing capacity, health system capacity; creation, distribution and procurement of treatments and vaccines, regulation of treatments, vaccines and health care, social support for vulnerable populations	Health actors can improve success in multi-stakeholder partnerships with sustainability goals; health actors can provide frameworks that help to understand complex problems with interconnected causality, e.g., One Health	The emergency nature of pandemic response can permit governance failures and corruption, e.g., human rights violations, graft, or other abuses of power. If pandemic response takes the form of highly centralized decisionmaking, stakeholders may be excluded from governance processes or be unable to participate in partnerships due to loss of needed resources
Access to science, technology and innovation	Access to treatments, vaccines, testing materials, emerging knowledge about virus	Healthy populations support scientific research and innovation; health sector supports research and development	The quality of global COVID-19 pandemic response affects which countries and populations have access to relevant science and technology, e.g., innovative treatments and vaccines
Data	Share up-to-date information on virus outbreaks, response strategies, vaccine and treatment efficacy, robust case and death records and population statistics vital for understanding the scale of the pandemic	Public health and health care sectors can support open data sharing and dissemination of knowledge	Data collection, analysis and dissemination related to pandemic response presents opportunities to continue these activities after the pandemic abates, with the risk that the needed resources to do so are withdrawn when the pandemic ends

response to the crisis, the reality of pandemic response at the global level has too often been economic and health nationalism rather than the multilateral and multisectoral cooperation envisioned in SDG17.

The COVID-19 pandemic, from its start, shows the interconnectedness of health and SDG17. COVID-19 was probably born of a specific food system (Box 13.1), was transmitted through the world via trade and travel linkages, and then showed the dependence of the international economy on health and health policies, both through the non-pharmaceutical interventions that drastically transformed countries in 2020 and through the importance of vaccine production and development.

First, the contribution of public health policy – in particular, One Health thinking – is visible in the origins and initial dissemination of the disease. The conditions under which the COVID-19 pandemic emerged highlight the need for sustainable development reforms to improve national and global food systems and protect the environment (see Box 13.1). A number of recent epidemics have been connected to zoonotic transmission. The ability for a contagious virus to cross over from an animal population to humans is connected to the sustainability of food supplies and how we interact with our environment, including how animals are kept, medically cared for, and transported, as well as related factors such as biodiversity loss and changing patterns of contact between wildlife, including insects, and humans. Whatever the origins of SARS-CoV-2, some of the underlying conditions that create opportunities for zoonotic transmission have not changed since the beginning of the pandemic. And due to the associated economic downturn, some may have worsened (WHO, 2021). The economic and health consequences of not addressing these conditions have been made crystal clear during the pandemic, making sustainable food supply chains a clear case of potential "co-benefits" – or potential "double disadvantages", outcomes which undermine both sustainable development and health. Including health professionals in discussions about agriculture, food sustainability and biodiversity, particularly those with expertise in environmental health, epidemiology and virology, will be essential in tackling the causes and consequences of zoonotic transmission of disease and its potential spillover into human populations. To avoid further outbreaks of this kind requires investment in strong and sustainable public health systems that can provide a regulatory approach that focuses directly on the consequences for human health, rather than a technocratic elaboration on existing trade policy, which is more likely to restrict trade without preventing future health crises (Lee & Houston, 2020).

Box 13.1 The case of COVID-19 and food systems

Emma Willoughby, University of Michigan

Following the speculation that COVID-19 emerged from a wet market in Wuhan, China, there has been renewed interest in the role of wildlife trade and zoonotic disease spillover. The wildlife trade purportedly generates immense wealth in places including Southeast Asia and Central Africa, and many point to the medicinal interests of those who practise traditional Chinese medicine as sources for increasing demand for wildlife meat and parts. However, there are other trade forces affecting wildlife trafficking and encouraging human settlement in forested areas.

In actuality, a majority of zoonoses emerge constantly and are not only linked back to wildlife markets. They are, however, connected to market forces. Some accounts attribute the 2003 SARS spillover to the wildlife markets themselves, but upstream this spillover first occurred between bats and intensive raising of palm-faced civets (McNamara et al., 2020). This story is similar to the emergence of Nipah virus from mainland Malaysia, where large pork farms were established bordering orchards which attracted large flying foxes (Breed et al., 2006). Pulliam and colleagues (2012) note that in particular, the intensive pork production provided an environment in which the virus could replicate and persist for years before leading to a full-scale outbreak.

In resource-rich countries where pressure to economically develop is high, there is demonstrable evidence that development brings settlement in closer proximity to wildlife. For example, researchers detail how mining and logging encampments expand to eventually form villages in areas that become fragmented forests, which are shown to support generalist species that may host a diversity of pathogens (Johnson et al., 2020; McNamara et al., 2020). Outbreaks of Ebolavirus variants have been linked to fruit bat encounters, and specifically bats which can survive in semi-domestic environments, not exclusively from bushmeat consumption (Marí Saéz et al., 2015). Rodents in mainland Southeast Asia have been shown to thrive in rice paddy environments and be a reservoir to a higher diversity of parasites (Bordes et al., 2013). Years of transformative agriculture and urbanization, land-use conversion and forest degradation all remain important contributors to zoonotic spillover (Bordes et al., 2013; Cui, Li & Shi, 2019; Jones et al., 2013). One Health is a collaborative approach incorporating the study and protection of human health, animal health and environmental health. Moving forward, researchers must consider the social transformations of the communities who are most vulnerable to economic demand and environmental stressors.

Second, while policy responses to the pandemic certainly reduced morbidity and mortality from the disease, they also shocked many economies. In terms of the elements of SDG17 that refer to finance, delivering a stable economic system, and trade, lockdown policies and fear of contagion dampened economic activity. Foreign Direct Investment (FDI) dropped in many countries during 2020 and 2021. Although the United Nations Conference on Trade and Development (UNCTAD) found that FDI recovered to pre-pandemic levels during 2022, the organization warned that the lingering effects of the pandemic, the war in Ukraine and climate disruption were likely to contribute to an ongoing poor investment climate (UNCTAD, 2022). This is particularly a concern for those countries which depend heavily on FDI, many of whom had been trying to increase investment as a development strategy prior to the pandemic. With less work for migrants in many places, and travel restrictions in place that often discriminated against non-nationals, remittances seem to have dwindled somewhat (although official statistics often did not reflect this decline as they do not track informal cash transfers) (Dinarte-Diaz, Jaume & Medina-Cortina, 2022; World Bank, 2022a). This was also most important in lower-income countries, where international remittances are a key source of income for many and can make up a significant proportion of GDP.

In terms of development finance specifically, concerns have been raised that many least developed countries (LDCs) are at risk of defaulting on their debt obligations, with the World Bank classifying over half as in debt distress or at risk of debt distress (World Bank, 2021a, 2022b). The pandemic was not the sole cause of this problem, but did exacerbate it. With the global economy in an uncertain state, interest rates and inflation ballooning, and many national economies shrinking rather than growing, debt distress becomes a much more significant concern. It is important to note that debt can be a consequence of a country trying to "develop" in sustainable ways, as sustainability requires infrastructure, which in turn requires investment. As FDI dwindles, private investment is not a substitute for public funds (Kharas & Dooley, 2021). Substantial debt relief will be needed in order to prevent countries in debt distress from defaulting, the consequences of which could be far-reaching and deliver a significant blow to any nascent recovery in the global economy (United Nations/DESA 2020). Debt relief could also, potentially, free up resources that could be invested in developing health systems, addressing both the pandemic and other ongoing, severe public health crises in poorer countries. From May 2020 until December 2021, debt relief was provided to eligible countries through the Debt Service Suspension Initiative (DSSI), but continuing provision was subject to the political will of high-income countries. The DSSI was highly criticized as ineffective, as it deferred rather than cancelled debt payments, it did not cover private sources of debt, and only 48 out of 73 eligible countries elected to participate (Bretton Woods Project, 2022; World Bank, 2021b). Historically, this form of limited debt relief has not solved the economic problems of poorer states. More than that, requirements to make regular payments and conditionality attached to debts has often prevented adequate investment in infrastructure such as health systems (Khan & Shanks, 2020).

In terms of trade specifically, keeping trade routes open is vital to pandemic response in terms of ensuring a stable flow of both routine goods as well as distribution of needed treatments and vaccines. In the early stages of the pandemic, disruptions attributable to the spread of the virus as well as pandemic response meant that states reliant on single commodities were left vulnerable to pandemic-related price shocks, while those that relied on trade for essential supplies such as food and medicines were heavily affected by COVID-related supply chain disruptions (Barlow et al., 2021). The volume of global trade shrank significantly in 2020 as production and consumption were scaled back. Trade volumes recovered surprisingly well in 2021, although this recovery faltered in 2022, and the outlook for 2023 is likely to be impacted by ongoing inflation and the war in Ukraine.

In terms of Overseas Development Assistance, a significant form of aid specifically addressed by SDG17, the picture is less clear, as ODA statistics are published on a long delay. Emerging data for 2020 suggest that health ODA for that year, while substantial overall and higher than prior years, may have shifted towards COVID concerns at the expense of ODA for basic health needs such as support for UHC and basic nutrition – the sorts of policies that are considered essential within the SDG framework for meeting states' health goals (Wallace Brown et al., 2022). And as national governments face budget constraints, it can be electorally more palatable to focus cuts in ways that affect people in other countries, making ODA a prime target. In 2021, the United Kingdom drastically cut the amount of ODA it provides to other countries, ending a longstanding policy of movement towards the internationally recognized 0.7% GDP target. Other countries may yet follow suit, with very concrete effects on health and wellbeing in lower-income countries that are still experiencing significant consequences from the pandemic.

The pandemic did not create many of these problems but has exacerbated existing vulnerabilities created by the global trade, investment and financial systems – existing vulnerabilities recognized in SDG17. The health sector can support sustainable economic growth and promote investment by providing necessary preventative, routine and emergency health care. Having a robust health sector with universal coverage lessens the burden of communicable and non-communicable disease on the whole of society with benefits for businesses and investors that include healthier and potentially more productive employees, fewer supply chain disruptions and fewer economic burdens relating to the provision of health coverage. Stronger health systems that could care for patients and administer vaccines, and social policy that could cushion the effects of NPIs clearly contributed to effective pandemic response (Greer et al., 2021a; Jarman, 2021).

Across trade, aid and finance, concerns are being raised that the pandemic experience and geopolitical tensions are creating pressure for states to become more isolationist, and move away from multilateral cooperation and multisectoral partnership as envisioned in SDG17. In several key areas of pandemic response, international cooperation has occurred, but has delivered mixed results. Vaccination against COVID-19 is a good illustration of this. In the early stages of the pandemic, rapid development of multiple effective vaccines for COVID-19 was a welcome surprise to many in the health sector (Saag, 2022). But distributing these vaccines was a different matter. As of February 2023, COVID-19 vaccines remain unaffordable and inaccessible for many low-income countries.

It was obvious long before the spread of COVID-19 that many countries would have to rely on international cooperation to deliver needed treatments and vaccines in the event of a large-scale pandemic (Fonseca et al., 2022). COVAX, for example, is a multilateral partnership between GAVI, CEPI and the WHO that was conceptualized as a means of ensuring the kind of multilateral, public–private cooperation enshrined in SDG17 in the area of COVID-19 vaccination. By 2022, COVAX had delivered a billion vaccine doses to 144 countries and territories, which is not a small feat. But here also, states acted in their own interests before acting to help others. Early in the pandemic, high-income countries purchased a significant portion of the global COVID-19 vaccine supply, able to buy in such bulk that their orders were prioritized by manufacturers. This left other states to rely more heavily on multilateral mechanisms like COVAX, which were relatively slow to disperse vaccines in the early stages of the pandemic, or on bilateral donations from other states, which were likely to come with strings attached and be limited by geopolitical concerns. Furthermore, some of the vaccines distributed with geopolitical intent were shown to be less effective than others. Comparing Serbia with Ukraine, for example, Serbia accepted vaccines from Russia and China to supplement its own supplies and also donated some of these supplies to neighbouring states. Russian and Chinese donations were not politically acceptable in Ukraine, however, which was left to rely on supplies from COVAX that were slow to arrive. As a result of these supply constraints, and prior to the war with Russia, Ukraine vaccinated a much lower proportion of its population and experienced one of the slowest vaccination rates in Europe.

A further set of issues centres around governance and multisectoral partnerships. In a number of countries, in fact in most countries in Europe, a study found that horizontal multisectoral collaboration in response to the pandemic was eschewed in favour of central control by the executive (Greer et al., 2021b, 2022b). A number of health experts and agencies, rather than being brought into key conversations about policy, were excluded from the process as authority was centralized. This happened as the political salience of the pandemic increased, with national leaders sometimes unwilling to delegate decisionmaking power to public health agencies and experts (Greer et al., 2022b). Actors in the health sector were often excluded from decisionmaking, with predictable results – the double disadvantage of renewed disease spread and protracted lockdown measures impacting economic growth.

A final set of questions during the pandemic arose around the availability of relevant technology and data. The pandemic was a huge test of progress towards these types of collaboration under SDG17. Communicable diseases do not respect national borders, and so publicly sharing key data on disease spread, the presence of variants, and population health outcomes cross-regionally and cross-nationally, in a timely manner, as well as open access to research on the disease, becomes very important. The ability to share key data internationally rests in part on the capacity within the health sector and government to gather and distribute data, as well as linguistic and technological barriers to interoperability. In a scenario where co-benefits are realized, health actors and the data they produce would facilitate policy decisionmaking on matters that affect not only health but also sustainable growth. In some places, this has occurred, with leaders making lockdown decisions based on available evidence. Regional, national and local public health agencies, non-profit organizations such as universities and think tanks, civil society groups, journalists and media outlets have all been central to promoting accessible data about the spread and effects of COVID-19, forming transnational, multisectoral partnerships. The presence of health actors in these partnerships is vital – they interpret data on disease spread and severity, evaluate treatments and vaccines, share research on new variants, formulate communications strategies and much more.

However, we can also point to examples of double disadvantages when it comes to sharing data. Some politicians have chosen to ignore relevant data, hoping the virus would go away, while others have actively suppressed access to information and sidelined health actors. In Brazil, for example, President Jair Bolsonaro sought to strongly downplay the impact of the pandemic. In June 2020, the Brazilian Ministry of Health removed public access to months of COVID-19 data, and ceased to publish the total number of confirmed cases (Mano, 2020). In the US state of Florida, data scientists employed by the state were pressured to manipulate COVID-19 statistics in ways that would downplay the impact of the virus and then asked to remove data from public view (NPR, 2020). In other cases, data have been framed in certain ways by individuals and groups working through media and social media channels, causing mis- and dis-information to proliferate. And in some places, a lack of investment in health infrastructure (for example, inadequate death registries, lack of testing or contact tracing, poor infrastructure for storing and sharing health data, few resources for public health messaging) hampers our ability to understand the true scale of the pandemic and compare pandemic responses cross-nationally. All of these factors have extended the pandemic; denialism and misinformation stoke vaccine hesitancy, increase distrust in governments, reduce compliance with public health measures and feed into poor policy decisionmaking. And the longer the pandemic runs, the greater its toll will be on economic growth.

13.4   Conclusion

SDG17 covers a broad range of policy areas that are considered vital in order to deliver on the other SDGs, including global economic stability and growth, the policies that fuel that growth, such as trade, aid and finance, multisectoral collaboration and governance, capacity building, and policies supporting access to science, technology and data. As this chapter shows, the co-benefits, or positive spillover effects between health and these other areas, are significant, and so are the potential negative spillover effects, or double disadvantages. The systems that support population health and wellbeing are a vital part of achieving sustainable development.

The COVID-19 pandemic has demonstrated the strong and important links between health, sustainability and the global economy, offering many examples of the essential role that health plays in making (co-benefits) or breaking (double disadvantages) progress towards SDG17. When health and sustainable growth goals align, good population health, resting on environmentally sustainable food chains, adequate support for public health systems, good access to health care, and good enough governance for health, can provide benefits to the global economy and help to move towards a model of sustainable development. Conversely, when population health is threatened – via the spread of communicable disease, increases in chronic conditions, poor access to health care, inadequate public health systems and underlying economic and social inequality – the goals of sustainable development can become unobtainable.

The COVID-19 pandemic shows, for example, how a widespread communicable disease can cause long-lasting economic disruption at a global scale as people withdraw from economic activity, and how the policy decisions adopted to control viral spread can impact the global economy. But it has also shown that the health sector, collaborating through multi-stakeholder partnerships that involve government finance and regulatory oversight, corporate and academic research, and global production chains, can deliver solutions – in this case, multiple safe and effective vaccines that protect against COVID-19, produced in record time. In turn, sound multilateral cooperation on key issues such as finance, trade, technology transfer and knowledge dissemination can provide the necessary funds to support health infrastructure in places where it is sorely needed. Building basic government capacity around vital records, data sharing, budgeting and revenue collection can also support key health systems and outcomes. In a virtuous circle, better health infrastructure can form a foundation for more sustainable growth.

Realizing this vision – the co-benefits from integrating SDG17 and health and avoiding the double disadvantages – requires some urgent and some ongoing actions. Urgently, high-income countries and other donors must deepen their commitment to providing much-needed debt relief and increase (rather than cut) international aid to address the ongoing economic and social consequences of the pandemic. And while actions to increase access to COVID-19 vaccines outside high-income countries ramped up in spring 2021, current global vaccine distribution remains inadequate to fully control spread and is not serving the poorest countries. In the longer term, the pandemic speaks to the need to invest in public health systems that can detect and counter disease and chronic conditions, as well as in comprehensive, universal access to health care, no matter the location. Failure to do this leaves the global economy vulnerable to future shocks and ongoing suboptimal outcomes.

Collaboration around SDG17 and health can provide significant co-benefits, or, as the pandemic has unfortunately demonstrated, a failure to collaborate can produce double disadvantages, outcomes which simultaneously worsen sustainable development and population health. It is very important that we learn the lessons of this pandemic as soon as possible, because they are also the lessons we need to learn to address ongoing inequality in the global economy through SDG17.

References

Acemoglu D, Johnson S (2007). Disease and Development: The Effect of Life Expectancy on Economic Growth. J Polit Econ, 115(6).

Addo-Atuah J, Senhaji-Tomza B, Ray D et al. (2020). Global health research partnerships in the context of the Sustainable Development Goals (SDGs). Res Soc Adm Pharm, 16(11):1614–1618. (https://doi.org/10.1016/j.sapharm.2020.08.015; Epub 2020 Aug 27. PMID: 32893133; PMCID: PMC7449894)

Alkire BC, Peters AW, Shrime MG et al. (2018). The Economic Consequences Of Mortality Amenable To High-Quality Health Care In Low- And Middle-Income Countries. Health Aff (Millwood), 37(6). (https://www.healthaffairs.org/doi/10.1377/hlthaff.2017.1233).

Barlow P, van Schalkwyk MCI, McKee M et al. (2021). COVID-19 and the collapse of global trade: building an effective public health response. Lancet Planet Health, 5(2):E102–107.

Boniol M, Kunjumen T, Nair TS et al. (2022). The global health workforce stock and distribution in 2020 and 2030: a threat to equity and "universal" health coverage? *BMJ Glob Health*, 7:e009316.

Bordes F, Herbreteau V, Dupuy S et al. (2013). The diversity of microparasites of rodents: a comparative analysis that helps in identifying rodent-borne rich habitats in Southeast Asia. Infect Ecol Epidemiology, 3:10.3402/iee.v3i0.20178. (https://doi.org/10.3402/iee.v3i0.20178)

Breed AC, Field HE, Epstein JH et al. (2006). Emerging henipaviruses and flying foxes – Conservation and management perspectives. Biol Conserv, 131(2):211–220. (https://doi.org/10.1016/j.biocon.2006.04.007).

Bretton Woods Project (2022). Ineffective G20 Debt Service Suspension Initiative ends as world faces worst debt crisis in decades. (https://www.brettonwoodsproject.org/2022/04/ineffective-debt-service-suspension-initiative-ends-as-world-faces-worst-debt-crisis-in-decades/)

Crosbie E, Defrank V, Egbe CO et al. (2021). Tobacco supply and demand strategies used in African countries. Bull World Health Organ, 99(7):539–540. (https://doi.org/10.2471/BLT.20.266932)

Cui J, Li F, Shi ZL (2019). Origin and evolution of pathogenic coronaviruses. Nat Rev Microbiol, 17:181–192. (https://doi-org.proxy.lib.umich.edu/10.1038/s41579-018-0118-9)

Dinarte-Diaz L, Jaume D, Medina-Cortina E (2022). Did remittances really increase during the pandemic? World Bank Blog, 11 July. (https://blogs.worldbank.org/developmenttalk/did-remittances-really-increase-during-pandemic).

Drope J, Lencucha R (2013). Tobacco control and trade policy: Proactive strategies for integrating policy norms. J Public Health Pol, 34:153–164. (https://doi.org/10.1057/jphp.2012.36)

Eurostat (2022). SDG 17 – Partnerships for the Goals. (https://ec.europa.eu/eurostat/statistics-explained/index.php?title=SDG_17_-_Partnerships_for_the_goals).

Evans RG, Barer ML, Marmor TR (eds). (1994). Why are some people healthy and others not?: The determinants of the health of populations. Transaction Publishers.

Friel S, Hattersley L, Snowdon W et al. (2013). INFORMAS. Monitoring the impacts of trade agreements on food environments. Obes Rev, 14(Suppl 1):120–134. (doi: 10.1111/obr.12081. PMID: 24074216)

GBD (2019). Diseases and Injuries Collaborators. The Global Burden of Disease Study. Lancet. (https://www.thelancet.com/infographics/gbd-2019)

GBD (2020). Diseases and Injuries Collaborators. Global burden of 369 diseases and injuries in 204 countries and territories, 1990–2019: a systematic analysis for the Global Burden of Disease Study 2019. Lancet Glob Health Metrics, 396(10258):P1204–1222. (https://doi.org/10.1016/S0140-6736(20)30925-9)

Greer SL, Jarman H, Falkenbach M et al. (2021a). Social policy as an integral component of pandemic response: learning from COVID-19 in Brazil, Germany, India, and the United States. Glob Public Health, 16(8–9):1209–1222.

Greer SL, King E, Massard da Fonseca E et al. (eds). (2021b). Coronavirus Politics. Ann Arbor, MI: University of Michigan Press.

Greer SL, Falkenbach M, Siciliani L et al. (2022a). From Health in All Policies to Health for All Policies. Lancet Public Health. (DOI: https://doi.org/10.1016/S2468-2667(22)00155-4)

Greer SL, Rozenblum S, Falkenbach M et al. (2022b). Centralizing and decentralizing governance in the COVID-19 pandemic: the politics of credit and blame. Health Policy, 126(5):408–417.

Gutiérrez-Hernández P, Abásolo-Alessón I (2021). The health care sector in the economies of the European Union: an overview using an input–output framework. Cost Eff Resour Alloc, 19(4). (https://doi.org/10.1186/s12962-021-00258-8)

Hughes RG, Lawrence MA (2005). Globalization, food and health in Pacific Island countries. Asia Pac J Clin Nutr, 14(4):298–306. (PMID: 16326635.)

Jarman H (2015). The Politics of Trade and Tobacco Control. Basingstoke, UK: Palgrave.

Jarman H (2017). Trade Policy Governance: What Health Policymakers and Advocates Need to Know. Health Policy, 121(11):1105–1112.

Jarman H (2019). Normalizing Tobacco? The Politics of Trade, Investment, and Tobacco Control. Milbank Q, 97(2):449–479. (doi: 10.1111/1468-0009.12393)

Jarman H (2021). State responses to the COVID-19 pandemic: governance, surveillance, coercion and social policy. In: Greer SL, King E, Massard da Fonseca E et al. (eds) Coronavirus Politics. Ann Arbor, MI: University of Michigan Press.

Jarman H, Koivusalo M (2017). Trade and health in the European Union. Research Handbook on EU Health Law and Policy, 429–452.

Johnson CK, Hitchens PL, Pandit PS et al. (2020). Global shifts in mammalian population trends reveal key predictors of virus spillover risk. Proc Royal Soc B, 287:2019273620192736. (http://doi.org/10.1098/rspb.2019.2736)

Jones BA, Grade D, Kock R et al. (2013). Zoonosis emergence linked to agricultural intensification and environmental change. Proc Natl Acad Sci USA, 110(21):8399–8404.

Khan M, Shanks S (2020). Decolonizing COVID-19: delaying external debt repayments. Lancet Glob Health (8)7:E897. (https://doi.org/10.1016/S2214-109X(20)30253-9)

Kharas H, Dooley M (2021). Debt distress and development distress: Twin crises of 2021. Brookings Institute Global Working Papers, 153 (March). (https://www.brookings.edu/wp-content/uploads/2021/03/Debt-distress-and-development-distress.pdf).

Koivusalo M (2014). Policy space for health and trade and investment agreements. Health Promot Int, 29(Suppl 1):i29–47. (doi: 10.1093/heapro/dau033. PMID: 25217355)

Lafferty W (1996). The politics of sustainable development: Global norms for national implementation, Env Polit, 5(2):185–208. (DOI: 10.1080/09644019608414261)

Leal Filho W, Wall T, Barbir J et al. (2022). Relevance of international partnerships in the implementation of the UN Sustainable Development Goals. Nat Commun, 13:613. (https://doi.org/10.1038/s41467-022-28230-x)

Lee A, Houston AR (2020). Diets, Diseases, and Discourse: Lessons from COVID-19 for Trade in Wildlife, Public Health, and Food Systems Reform. Food Ethics, 5:17. (https://doi.org/10.1007/s41055-020-00075-4)

Lee K, Carpenter C, Challa C et al. (2009). The strategic targeting of females by transnational tobacco companies in South Korea following trade liberalisation. Global Health, 5:2. (https://doi.org/10.1186/1744-8603-5-2)

Maani N, Petticrew M, Galea S (eds) (2022). The Commercial Determinants of Health. Oxford: OUP.

Maani N, Collin J, Friel S et al. (2020). Bringing the commercial determinants of health out of the shadows: a review of how the commercial determinants are represented in conceptual frameworks. Eur J Public Health, 30(4):660–664.

McGrady B (2011). Trade and Public Health: The WTO, Tobacco, Alcohol, and Diet. Cambridge: Cambridge University Press.

MacKenzie R, Collin J (2012). Trade policy, not morals or health policy: The US Trade Representative, tobacco companies and market liberalization in Thailand. Glob Soc Policy, 12(2):149–172. (doi:10.1177/1468018112443686)

McNamara J, Robinson E, Abernethy K et al. (2020). COVID-19, Systemic Crisis, and Possible Implications for the Wild Meat Trade in Sub-Saharan Africa. Environ Resour Econ, 1–22. Advance online publication. (https://doi.org/10.1007/s10640-020-00474-5)

Mano A (2020). Brazil takes down COVID-19 data, hiding soaring death toll. Reuters, 6 June. (https://www.reuters.com/article/us-health-coronavirus-brazil/brazil-takes-down-covid-19-data-hiding-soaring-death-toll-idUSKBN23D0PW)

Marí Saéz A, Weiss S, Nowak K et al. (2015). Investigating the zoonotic origin of the West African Ebola epidemic. EMBO Mol Med, 7(1):17–23. (https://doi.org/10.15252/emmm.201404792).

Marmot M, Allen J (2014). Social determinants of health equity. Am J Public Health, 104(S4):S517–S519.

Marmot M, Allen J, Goldblatt P et al. (2010). Fair Society, Healthy Lives. Institute of Health Equity. (https://www.instituteofhealthequity.org/resources-reports/fair-society-healthy-lives-the-marmot-review)

Marmot M, Allen J, Boyce T et al. (2020). Marmot Review – 10 Years On. Institute of Health Equity. (https://www.instituteofhealthequity.org/resources-reports/marmot-review-10-years-on).

Massard da Fonseca E, Jarman H, King EJ et al. (2022). Perspectives in the study of the political economy of COVID-19 vaccine regulation. Regul Gov, 16(4):1283–1289.

Mitlin D (1992). Sustainable development: a guide to the literature. Environ Urban, 4(1):111–124.

NPR (2020). Florida Scientist Says She Was Fired For Not Manipulating COVID-19 Data. NPR Morning Edition, 29 June. (https://www.npr.org/2020/06/29/884551391/florida-scientist-says-she-was-fired-for-not-manipulating-covid-19-data)

Oliveira-Duarte L, Aparecida Reis D, Fleury AL, (2021). Innovation Ecosystem framework directed to Sustainable Development Goal #17 partnerships implementation. Sustainable Development 29(5):1018–1036. (https://doi.org/10.1002/sd.2191)

Pulliam JR, Epstein JH, Dushoff J et al. (2012). Agricultural intensification, priming for persistence and the emergence of Nipah virus: a lethal bat-borne zoonosis. J R Soc Interface, 9(66):89–101. (https://doi.org/10.1098/rsif.2011.0223)

Remes J, Linzer K, Singhal S et al. (2020). Prioritizing Health: A Prescription for Prosperity. McKinsey and Company Special Report. (https://www.mckinsey.com/industries/healthcare-systems-and-services/our-insights/prioritizing-health-a-prescription-for-prosperity).

Saag M (2022). Wonder of wonders, miracle of miracles: the unprecedented speed of COVID-19 science. Physiol Rev, 102(3):1569–1577. (doi: 10.1152/physrev.00010.2022. Epub 2022 Apr 21. PMID: 35446679; PMCID: PMC9169823)

Sachs J (2015). The Age of Sustainable Development. Columbia University Press.

Shaffer ER, Brenner JE, Houston TP (2005). International trade agreements: a threat to tobacco control policy. Tob Control, 14:ii19–ii25.

Sharma R (2018). Health and economic growth: Evidence from dynamic panel data of 143 years. PLoS One, 13(10):e0204940. (https://doi.org/10.1371/journal.pone.0204940)

Skrzypek K (2020). Trade in pharmaceuticals and medical goods in 2019 and COVID-19 implications for 2020. (https://ihsmarkit.com/research-analysis/trade-in-pharmaceuticals-and-medical-goods-in-2019-and-covid19.html).

Snowdon W, Thow AM (2013). Trade policy and obesity prevention: challenges and innovation in the Pacific Islands. Obes Rev, 14(Suppl 2):150–158. (doi: 10.1111/obr.12090. PMID: 24102909)

Thow AM, Swinburn B, Colagiuri S et al. (2010). Trade and food policy: Case studies from three Pacific Island countries, Food Policy, 35(6):556–564. (https://doi.org/10.1016/j.foodpol.2010.06.005)

UNCTAD (2022). World Investment Report 2022. (https://unctad.org/publication/world-investment-report-2022)

United Nations (2018). Review of SDGs Implementation: SDG 17 – Strengthening the means of implementation and revitalize the global partnership for sustainable development. (https://sustainabledevelopment.un.org/index.php?menu=2993&nr=4163&page=view&type=20000)

United Nations (2022). SDG 17: Targets and Indicators. (https://sdgs.un.org/goals/goal17)

United Nations/DESA (2020). COVID and Sovereign Debt. Policy Briefs 72. (https://www.un.org/development/desa/dpad/publication/un-desa-policy-brief-72-covid-19-and-sovereign-debt/)

Wallace Brown G, Tacheva B, Shahid M et al. (2022). Global health financing after COVID-19 and the new Pandemic Fund. Brookings Institute, 7 December. (https://www.brookings.edu/blog/future-development/2022/12/07/global-health-financing-after-covid-19-and-the-new-pandemic-fund/)

Weber H, Weber M (2020). When means of implementation meet Ecological Modernization Theory: A critical frame for thinking about the Sustainable Development Goals initiative. World Dev, 136:105129. (https://doi.org/10.1016/j.worlddev.2020.105129)

WHO (2021). WHO-convened Global Study of the Origins of SARS-CoV-2. (https://www.who.int/health-topics/coronavirus/origins-of-the-virus)

WHO Commission on Social Determinants of Health (2008). Final Report. (http://apps.who.int/iris/bitstream/handle/10665/43943/9789241563703_eng.pdf;jsessionid=3A7FB69DBC6EE5C2D967C2DBD4CC95DF?sequence=1)

Williams GA, Jacob G, Rakovac I et al. (2020). Health professional mobility in the WHO European Region and the WHO Global Code of Practice: data from the joint OECD/EUROSTAT/WHO-Europe questionnaire, Eur J Public Health, 30(Suppl 4):iv5–iv11. (https://doi.org/10.1093/eurpub/ckaa124)

Wismar M, Maier CB, Glinos IA et al. (eds). (2011). Health Professional Mobility and Health Systems: Evidence from 17 European Countries.

Copenhagen: World Health Organization/European Observatory on Health Systems and Policies.

World Bank (2021a). Debt Sustainability Analysis. (https://www.worldbank .org/en/programs/debt-toolkit/dsa)

World Bank (2021b). COVID-19: Debt Service Suspension Initiative. (https:// www.worldbank.org/en/topic/debt/brief/covid-19-debt-service-suspension-initiative)

World Bank (2022a). Neither by Land nor by Sea : The Rise of Electronic Remittances during COVID-19 (English). Policy Research working paper WPS 10057; COVID-19 (Coronavirus). Washington, DC: World Bank Group. (http://documents.worldbank.org/curated/en/099434205232231209/ IDU0b9463f130c07f040160bb26018c9daadd997)

World Bank (2022b). When the debt crises hit, don't simply blame the pandemic. World Bank Blogs, 28 June. (https://blogs.worldbank.org/voices/ when-debt-crises-hit-dont-simply-blame-pandemic)

Yamey G (2002). Have the latest reforms reversed WHO's decline? BMJ (Clinical research ed.), 325(7372):1107–1112. (https://doi.org/10.1136/ bmj.325.7372.1107)

Index

For EU product safety concerns, contact us at Calle de José Abascal, 56–1°, 28003 Madrid, Spain or eugpsr@cambridge.org.

www.ingramcontent.com/pod-product-compliance
Ingram Content Group UK Ltd.
Pitfield, Milton Keynes, MK11 3LW, UK
UKHW050735090126
466816UK00020B/394